True

Beauty

Emme

with Daniel Paisner

A Perigee Book

True Beauty

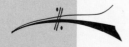

Positive Attitudes

and Practical Tips from

the World's Leading

Plus-Size Model

Most Perigee Books are available at special quantity discounts for bulk purchases for sales promotions, premiums, fund-raising, or educational use. Special books, or book excerpts, can also be created to fit specific needs.

For details, write: Special Markets, The Berkley Publishing Group, 200 Madison Avenue, New York, New York 10016.

A Perigee Book
Published by The Berkley Publishing Group
A member of Penguin Putnam Inc.
200 Madison Avenue
New York, NY 10016

G. P. Putnam's Sons edition: January 1997
First Perigee edition: March 1998
Perigee ISBN: 0-399-52383-9

Published simultaneously in Canada

The Penguin Putnam Inc. World Wide Web site address is
http://www.penguinputnam.com

The Library of Congress has catalogued the G. P. Putnam's Sons edition as follows:

Emme.
    True beauty : positive attitudes and practical tips from the world's leading plus-size model / Emme with Daniel Paisner.
        p.   cm.
    Includes bibliographical references.
    ISBN 0-399-14204-5
    1. Beauty, personal.   2. Overweight women—Psychology.
3. Body image.   4. Body size—Psychological aspects.
5. Self-esteem in women.   6. Emme.   7. Models—
United States—Biography.   I. Paisner, Daniel.   II. Title.
RA778.E52   1996   96-44351 CIP
646.7'042—dc21

Printed in the United States of America

10   9   8   7   6   5   4   3   2   1

Acknowledgments

I must have had a little angel sitting on my shoulder over the last couple of years, namely because of some very special people who heard my message, believed in it and took action.

My publicist, Sarah Hall, provided the door that led to the making of this book. I thank you for your incredible insight, unmatchable work savvy and friendship . . . Mikal St. George, thank you for your assistance . . . I had no idea what it would take to write a book, but thanks to my dear friend and literary agent, Dan Strone, of the William Morris Agency, who believed in me and encouraged me to share my story, this is now a reality. I couldn't have done it without you. Many thanks to Debra Bard ... Dan Paisner—I thank you for being such a wonderful person to work with over the last year. You pushed me, made me go beyond rewrite after rewrite and made the sea of ideas and emotions come together in a book that makes me very proud ... Stacy Creamer, editor extraordinaire, you developed this book into a living, breathing and inspiring reality, right down to the wire! I thank you, and the rest of the Putnam gang, for your commitment and confidence in me.

To my family: Aunt Jessica and Aunt B., thank you for your neverending faith, love and wisdom . . . Chip and Mel, for listening, sharing and not being afraid of growing; I am so proud of you both . . . Jen, Jen, you're the best! . . . Judy (my opinionated and valued manuscript reader) and Herm, thank you for loving me as your own and being there when I need you most ... Jonathan, you've given me the gift of showing what courage is all about; God blessed you with your miracle ... Seth, Liora, Arianna and Benjamin, I love you all so much and appreciate all the support in everything I do . . . Granny and Gramps, for being the loving grandparents I never had . . . Marlene, thank God for you . . . Cousin Morty ("Shit or get off the pot!"), thank you . . .

Frank and Heurta and Uncle Walter, for your love and always open ear; thank you for being at every turn . . . And Bill, I wish only good and healthy things for you . . . I thank you all for making me the person I am today.

A special thanks to Danny and Lois Laitman, Mark and Amy Fierro, Roz Lichter, Andy Siegel, Eric Offner, Eric Zohn, Larry and Caroline Tedesco, Brian Dubin and his team, I am so glad to have you on *my* team . . . to Patty Sicular, my friend and number-one booker, to the Fords and all my bookers, thank you for a wonderful career . . . to Rosemary O'Brien, for all your help . . . to Staś, for shooting anytime, anywhere . . . Sergio, Fergie, Janice, Adam G., Adam W., Josh (d.n.), Jill G., Evans in London, C. W. Blume, Jacci, Suzanne V., Jerri and Kim Johnston, thank you! . . . to Victor M. Fornari and Shawn Frank of North Shore University Hospital's Center for Eating Disorders, and to the patients who so generously shared their thoughts and experiences . . . to Juliette Taska for an intuition ahead of her time . . . to Elizabeth Weinstock, Ph.D., and Jane Shure, Ph.D., for their studies on overcoming shame, and to the OMEGA Institute, ANAD and EDAP, for all that you've done for millions of people . . . to Lisa Berzins, Ph.D., executive director of P.L.E.A.S.E., for pushing legislation . . . to Alice Fornari, of Long Island

University's Center for Nutrition on the C.W. Post campus, for your patience and insight . . . and to all the women who opened their hearts, I can't thank you enough for your passion. I got the message.

There is no way I could mention each and every person who helped me get to this point in my life; I simply wouldn't have enough room, so let me say a heartfelt thank you to my loving friends and family who made a difference, gave me their time and opened their homes when I needed them over the years.

Since the original publication of this book, I have met countless generous people from all over the country and the world who provided me with a home away from home during the many months on the road. They helped to make this often lonely experience one that was inspiring and thrilling.

I want to thank my Perigee publisher, John Duff, and his wonderful staff for helping me make this paperback edition an even better way to touch people.

I've saved the best for last . . . To my husband, Phillip; your constant support, love and nonstop helping out were essential to my accomplishing this goal. Each day we love, we share, we grow, I am so blessed to have you in my life. Thank you for always being there.

God, through you all things are made possible. Thank you.

I dedicate this book to my mother, Sally, and the many women who battle with their body image and self-confidence today. May you find peace in the fact that you are not alone.

Contents

Contents

1

Take a
Second Look

*"All that you are is a result of
all that you have thought."*
—Buddha

In retrospect, I can see it was a case of right place,
right timing.

I was tooling around in my 1978 Oldsmobile,
trying to cram a month's worth of errands into my
one free afternoon, when I pulled up at a red light
near our local junior high school. I had the radio on,
but I don't remember what was playing. I don't even
recall what the weather was like or where, precisely,
I was headed. I sat in my car, idling at a school cross-
ing I passed through nearly every day when I was in
town.

Through the passenger-side window I saw a young

girl trudging to school carrying a six-pack of a brand-name diet drink at her hip. We're not talking diet sodas here, but those chalky nutritional supplements marketed by pharmaceutical companies and endorsed by ex-jocks and soap opera actresses. This girl walked with the cool assurance of someone twice her age, swinging that six-pack as if it was a point of pride, and at first it didn't strike me as any sort of big deal.

But the red light was a long one so I did a double take and really checked this girl out. There was something about her . . . She looked to be in good shape, possibly even athletic. She was a big girl, large for her age but with a shape that looked strong rather than fat. She was about thirteen, with a gorgeous mane of jet-black hair and breasts her girlfriends could only envy.

Okay, so those diet drinks said she was concerned about her weight. So were a lot of kids. So was I. To tell you the truth, when she turned her head I might have seen myself in her eyes. That was me! All those years ago!

As a teenager, I was bigger than all my friends— taller, rounder, fuller, heavier—and extremely self-conscious because of it. Like me, this girl was born with a large frame. She would never have the impossibly slim figure of the classic runway models, but she certainly wasn't fat. She was like a million other average- to large-sized kids—trying desperately to fit in, to look like the girls in the magazine ads, to be something she was not. But at what cost?

Those diet drinks she was carting around might be "doctor recommended," but what the advertising neglects to mention is that they were initially designed as a diet supplement for patients recovering from surgery, those with gastrointestinal problems and cancer patients undergoing chemotherapy. They are not a healthy substitute for a balanced diet—especially not for a thirteen-year-old who should be chewing her meals, not sipping them through a straw.

Looking at this girl, I couldn't help but wonder how much of her energies were focused on achieving a figure that would be difficult, if not impossible, for her to attain, given her body type, and to what lengths she was willing to go in that attempt to achieve it.

I wanted to get out of the car and shake some sense into this girl. I also had a lot of questions for her. Did being thin matter to her so very much? How long had she been concerned about her weight? Had our culture reached the point where the struggle to be thin began before adolescence?

But I let the moment pass. When the light finally turned green I tried to refocus on the rest of my day and pulled away, but as I drove on I couldn't shake the issues seeing that girl had raised in my mind.

I never chug-a-lugged diet supplements when I was her age back in the early 1970s, but only because they weren't widespread at the time. Had they been more available I have no doubt I would have sucked them back big time. My weight had always been a problem, and I went through periods where I would have done just about anything to look more like my slimmer, daintier friends.

So even though I saw so much of myself in this girl, I let her go on about her business like it was none of mine, at a time when I was uniquely positioned to reach out to her. I was one of the hardest-working models in the full-figured division at Ford Models. (Plus-size modeling is the fastest-growing segment of the modeling industry, helping to sell women's fashions size fourteen and up.) According to my press clippings I had reached the very top of my field. I was five feet eleven inches, about one hundred ninety pounds and, after a lot of physical and emotional work, I finally felt sensational about myself even at such an "unfashionable" size. I'd grown up thinking that my body was somehow my enemy and now that same body was helping me to earn a very comfortable living. I still didn't fit any mainstream notions of beauty, but I felt great and even though

I was in a profession that valued external beauty, I'd come to know that true beauty came from inside.

This was no small revelation. I had spent my entire childhood and much of my young adulthood grappling with weight and body-consciousness issues. Now I was living proof that it wasn't your dress size that matters. What matters is your health. Are your talents being put to use? Are you content? Could you consider yourself happy?

It would be ludicrous to argue that looks don't matter. After all, appearances are the first thing we have to go on when we meet someone new. And while we can work on those appearances, it's even more important to work on our inner selves. But more on that later . . .

I had a lot to say to this diet drink–guzzling teenager. Back in junior high school, I went through enough Tab to know what muscles get developed carting around six-packs like that. I'd gone on my share of fad diets, and cheated on all of them. I'd struggled my way into bathing suits one size too small. I counted calories and fat grams and watched the clock between meals. I worried if guys would want to go out with me when I was bigger than they were. As a kid, I was made to recognize that no meal was without cost. And yet here I was, at the other end of it all, a survivor. Hell, I wasn't just surviving,

I was thriving. And lucky for me, I wasn't the only one who felt more than okay about myself. Top fashion clients paid me good money to wear their clothes. I was working with some of the best photographers, stylists and makeup artists, all over the world. This moment back home in New Jersey was really nothing more than a pit stop, a chance to refuel and get my errands out of the way before jetting off to another assignment in an exotic locale.

I'm not a superstitious person, but I don't believe in coincidence either. Some things are just meant to be; sometimes just the right person is put in your path at a critical time. But if I was placed near this thirteen-year-old girl's path for a reason, I didn't get close enough. I didn't stop, didn't talk to her. Maybe I thought I was being polite, or that I didn't have time, or that the girl wouldn't be receptive to a stranger like me, but I chose not to get involved.

I thought about that girl all day, and for weeks afterward. I think about her still, and I imagine how our conversation might have gone. Really, I've replayed that moment over and over. I'd like to think that if I had a chance to see her again I would stop. I would take the time to find out what's up with her, what she's feeling, what she thinks. I've thought a lot about what I would try to say to her, how to share some of my experience—*without* sounding preachy.

After all, all our journeys sound easier in retrospect, as if the destination was always sure. It's taken a lot of thinking and some research, but I've finally been able to articulate the kind of message I would like to share with a girl like the one I saw that day and with the many millions of other women who fall outside of the currently "ideal" thin-body type.

I'd like to tell them that it's okay to be a bit outside the curve. Go ahead and cast a bigger shadow, but make sure you're healthy and fit and happy. Make sure you take the time to eat right, and eat smart. Set some goals for what you want out of this life and work to get there. Know that nearly anything you want is there for the taking. Ask yourself if your lifestyle is helping you or getting in your way. Our self-esteem doesn't have to take a body blow just because we're fuller and rounder than the girl on the cover of *Cosmo*. Success, health, happiness, beauty . . . they come in all shapes and sizes, for all people.

We are all built differently, and yet every woman I know has at one time or another tried to fit herself into some perverse notion of what she should look like. What a waste!

If the image-makers and pharmaceutical companies and fashion designers have their way we will always be made to feel like we don't fit. Either we don't fit the clothes, or we don't fit the ideal, or we don't fit the lifestyle. We just don't fit, period. It's a shame, it really is. We're being sold on an image of the super-thin, super-fit supermodel, but that's not who we are, not by a couple of dress sizes. Just flip back to the cover of this book and you'll see it's not who I am. If you've read this far, it's probably not who you are either.

It's certainly easy to say, Accept your size. Cast a bigger shadow. Be healthy, fit and happy. You may be thinking, Gee, I might as well go ahead and win the lottery too! Well, I don't mean to sound casual. From personal experience, I know the road to self-esteem can be a long one, full of detours and dead ends. So rather than have me tell you what you should do, let me tell you what happened to me. You may not identify with all of the particulars of my story, but I think you'll connect with the feelings. And when you do, you'll know you're not alone. And it's not just you and me. Sixty percent of American women wear dresses size twelve and up. That means, at a minimum, sixty percent of American women are not fitting the culture's body image. I leave it to you to figure what percentage of us can measure our unhappiness by how far we are from that ideal. I can tell you honestly this is no longer my measure of unhappiness, though it was for many years. For most of my youth and early adulthood, trying to shape my body to that ideal—an ideal wholly inappropriate for my body type—occupied more of my waking moments than any other single thing. This is not a fact I am proud of, but it is a fact. Between dieting, fasting, cheating on diets, breaking fasts, sneak binges, counting calories or grams of fat, and exercise, much of my life was devoted to beating myself up for overeating and fear of the overeating demon. I was pursuing an ideal that was unattainable—or at best an ideal whose price was far too high in terms of health, sanity and effort.

There is an alternative. And no, that alternative isn't giving yourself permission to be obese. As I sometimes tell people who say to me, "You're not fat," I am not the model for obesity. I am a plus-size model, a model for a size and shape that is not today's preferred norm, even though it is by far the norm; more women are closer to my size than Kate Moss's. What I'm advocating is an acceptance of that size—by the culture but, more important, by women like us: women whose natural body type is at variance with the culture's ideal. I like being out there in the media—in ads in newspapers and magazines, most recently on a billboard in Times Square (the first time a model of our size made it to such famed real estate).

"Fine for you," you may say, "you're a top model."

But as I'll explain, self-esteem is what makes a woman beautiful, and self-esteem has to radiate from within. That's true for women (and men!) of any size. I do believe, however, that because of the way our culture prizes a certain immaculately thin body type, fuller-figured women face particular impediments to genuine self-esteem because by society's lights, by definition, we're too big, too large, too round and too heavy to be desirable. It's tough to buck the culture, but it can be done, little by little. We can learn not to fall prey to the idealistic body image of the moment, to look beyond the cloudy haze to a life waiting to be fully lived. I'm hoping that I can help to erode the ultra-slim monolith every time I'm featured in an ad. But that's not enough. It's time I articulate the message. I didn't take the chance to do so when I was stopped at that light by that thirteen-year-old girl, but I'm hoping to make up for that now. If I'm right, and there are no coincidences, maybe she'll be reading this someday too . . .

2

The Start
of Something

My earliest memories have nothing to do
with the way I looked. It's weird, but for
someone whose young adult life was col-
ored by an uncertain body image, my childhood was
fairly idyllic—and fat-free, at least in the sense that
our house was nowhere near as "fat focused" as it
would become. Weight was hardly an issue; the bathroom scale was for gathering dust in the closet; mir-
rors were for making funny faces; meals were an
excuse to practice our table manners.

My mother and I lived in New York then, just the
two of us, in a two-bedroom apartment on the

Upper East Side. It was a glorious, innocent time, although I realize now what a struggle it must have been for my mother. I treasured the unique way we lived, and the us-against-the-world perspective that came with it. The only families even remotely like ours were on television.

My mother was the bravest lady in Manhattan, maybe even in the whole world. She was divorced, and worked two jobs. She had lived about a dozen lives. Her maiden name was Sally Lamar Owens, and I thought she had the perfect childhood. She was born in Trinidad, raised in Italy and Egypt, and sent to school in Switzerland. My grandfather worked for Standard Oil, so Mom hopscotched with her family from one exotic place to the next, soaking up all these different ways of being and seeing and doing.

"Melissa," she used to say, long before she abandoned my given name for my girlhood nickname, Em, "you can't imagine."

But she was wrong. I could. And I did. Often.

Even as a child, I marveled at Mom's unusual life. That, and how beautiful she was. I know most kids have a distorted image of their parents, but my mother truly was beautiful. I have the pictures to prove it. She was tall, about five feet ten inches, with a nice, large frame, a shapely figure and stunning auburn highlights to her long brown hair. She had the most enormous smile. She had large feet, which she always thought were ungainly, though they never bothered me. And she smelled great—just the right amount of just the right perfume, mixed with just the right amount of her. I wanted to stay inside her hugs for a long, long time.

My father also cut a striking figure, although to a little girl living in a different house it was not always the most agreeable one. His name was Tom Miller, and he was like a giant to me, almost untouchable. I never put him on the same pedestal as my mother, but he didn't need one. He was about six feet seven inches, and extremely handsome. He had blond hair, an athletic build and the deepest voice I'd ever heard. (He also had big feet, so I might have known what I was in for!) Unfortunately, he was kind of clueless as a father. He always told me he loved me, and I'm sure he did, but he didn't quite know how to show it.

My parents divorced when I was still an infant, so from my earliest memories on it was just me and Mom. She was my mother *and* father. She was my very best friend. She'd come home from work, and I'd be fed and bathed and ready for bed, and I'd run to meet her at the door just like other kids would run to meet their fathers. She always had a treat for me hidden in one of her pockets—a Chuckle, or some other candy—and the game was I'd have to search through her checkered wool coat to find it. We'd laugh, and tell each other about our days, and pick a book off the shelf to read before bed. Sometimes I'd put on one of my little costumes—a tutu, or an Indian headdress—and do a little star turn for her. I remember thinking that the rest of the world fell away the moment she walked through the door. Whatever stories I had to tell my mother were wonderful, whatever drawings I made were the best she'd ever seen, whatever skills I had mastered during the day were no match for her. I was, she said, God's little gift, and she showered me with unconditional love and praise.

Life, for this only child of a broken marriage, was pretty good.

Enter Bill, a man who would have me calling him Dad before the year was out. Now, I don't mean to give this man such an ominous introduction, but in looking back I can't shake thinking that our lives changed color on his arrival. I know mine did, and it had to do with how he influenced the way I looked out at the world and the way I began to believe the rest of the world looked back at me. I went from being the center of my mother's universe to a self-conscious kid who was never good enough.

Bill doted on me at first. He was a high-school

band instructor. He was tall, like my father, about six feet six inches, and he must have weighed over three hundred pounds. He was such an immense physical presence that next to him even a formidable, courageous woman like my mother seemed to shrink. One day, she was absolutely in charge, and the next she was dancing around the apartment, singing songs about her new "Mr. Right." Within weeks, they were making plans to marry. It all happened so fast.

We moved to a little log cabin in West Milford, New Jersey. I loved that house, and I loved those first few months with Bill, too. (It was the first time I ever got to play in snow!) He was like a real father to me. He taught me to fish. He built me a great tree house, and he set out all kinds of things for me to play with in our new backyard. It was great. In New York, I'd known only concrete playgrounds and structured outings in the park, but here I was free to explore, and dream. The tree house was hardly more than a platform, but it was my special hideaway. There were kids around, but I didn't have any close friends. It was just me and my little house in the woods.

Bill did a lot of nice things for me, early on. He taught me to cook, and to dance. One of my favorite things was to dance in his arms; his size made me feel so safe. He passed on his love for music, which was probably his most precious gift. But there was also a dark side to Bill, and he showed that too. He had had an unhappy childhood we were not supposed to ask about. He had children he rarely saw from another marriage. He had a temper. And he had a weight problem that would prove to be destructive to his health, and to the health of our family.

The temper showed itself first. Once, a few months into our new routine, he became so out of control during an argument with my mother that he punched a hole through a wall. It was like something out of a movie, but the terror I felt was real. At the time, my mother was pregnant with my brother, Chip, and as I recoiled at the thud and the tumbling bits of plasterboard I tried to catch Mom's eye for some reassurance that everything was going to be okay. Who was this man who wanted me to call him Dad? What had she gotten us into? Was it too late to go back to how we were? Mom may have been having second thoughts, but she never said anything. She truly loved this man, and accepted him as he was: warm and cuddly one minute, cold and unreachable (or explosive) the next.

Bill was an over-the-top disciplinarian, and my mother was anxious to support him in his authority. Mom knew how confused I was about Bill's entry into our life and the abrupt changes that ensued; she always came into my room to help me understand

Bill's position and I usually cried about how much things had changed, about how I wanted our old life back.

Bill did have his moments. He could be so sweet, and so kind, and then there was this other side to him that was like a tornado. He'd storm around the house for just a few minutes and I'd steel myself and think, *Okay, it's gonna be okay.* But it never was.

After a while, Mom thought a change of scenery might help. She found an ad for a junior-high-school music instructor at the Aramco oil company compound in Dhahran, Saudi Arabia, and encouraged Bill to apply. It was, we all thought, a too-perfect fit. For me, it was the chance to live the kind of exotic fairy tale of my mother's childhood, to experience what she had, to be more like her. I'm sure underneath our shared expectations was the silent hope that there would be less pressure on Bill in this new setting, that he would find a way to calm his violent mood swings and settle into his more nurturing mode.

There was a lot to do before taking off. I was only seven or eight, but I knew that we were going on a very long plane ride, to the middle of a desert, to a place where it was very, very hot. I knew that the oil company somehow produced the gasoline that made our cars run. I knew the people there would speak a different language, and that they would dress differently and think differently and behave differently. I knew Bill would teach music and band in an English-language school for children of oil company employees, the same school that I would attend. And I knew that our lives would never be the same.

We had to pack—not just our clothes but our entire household. Mom's crystal and silver, her antiques, the few pieces of furniture she and Bill had bought together . . . we were taking everything. The movers showed up one afternoon with a gigantic container, about the size of our living room, and in just a few hours they emptied our house into it.

One travel memory stands out. On the way to John F. Kennedy Airport, Bill had the taxi driver stop at a Carvel ice cream place in Queens. He had been talking about this "treat" for weeks, and now here it was. We all got out of the car and piled inside. "Melissa," he said, placing a jumbo sundae with hot fudge and whipped cream and nuts and three kinds of ice cream on the table in front of me, "you're not gonna get one of these for a long time, so you better eat up." He had one for himself, and one for my mother. I can still see us sitting there, underneath the rumble of jets flying in and out of JFK, the meter running on the cab outside, inhaling these killer ice cream sundaes like it was our last supper.

This pre-takeoff episode at the Carvel epitomizes the obsession, the love-hate relationship with food that Bill introduced to our household. Think about it. At this time, ice cream was never allowed in our home. Sweets of any kind were doled out sparingly, if at all. I went to school with my "Partridge Family" lunch box packed with good-for-you snacks and sandwiches that no kid would want to trade for. I'd watch as my friends swapped their Fluffernutter sandwiches and Scooter Pies, usually sitting by myself at the far end of the cafeteria to avoid their teasing. Through it all, the message was clear: Sweets and comparable indulgences were strictly forbidden. Yet there we were at that Carvel, scarfing down ice cream sundaes as if this was our last meal before our execution. And Bill had been talking up this splurge for weeks.

I don't mean to make too much of this, but consider the choices our family might have made in terms of our last big shindig in the United States before an overseas exodus that might keep us away from our country for years. Some father might have taken the family to the Statue of Liberty or the Empire State Building. Maybe a Broadway show or an amusement park. But Bill took us for a much anticipated ice cream binge.

I don't think this Carvel incident caused my troubled patterns of eating that developed later on, but it is emblematic of the attitude toward food that informed so much of my thinking. I can still remember the desperation in that outing far more than the joy. There was a get-it-while-you-can feeling about it, and definitely the notion that more had to be better, particularly since we didn't know how long we would have to do without. I look back and see myself shoveling in the ice cream and I know how clearly I got that message: You may deny yourself this pleasure on a daily basis—deny yourself, police yourself, resist temptation—but no matter how long you do without, this is what you really want. And every now and then, to reward yourself or console yourself, or to tide yourself over when you know you'll have to do without, you can let yourself go on one wild, uncontrolled binge.

The gust of hot, humid air when we stepped onto the tarmac at Dhahran was nothing that anyone could have prepared me for. Everyone had been saying it would be like a sauna. They told us it would be hot, but this was wild. It was difficult to breathe at first. Even the ground was hot, like the top of a stove. The absolutely strangest thing was the way the Arabs looked at me, almost from the moment I stepped off the plane. I was a stocky, tow-headed tomboy, with short hair and pale skin. I'd never really thought about how I looked, and now I couldn't not think about it. The locals had no frame of reference for someone like me, and I felt like the main attraction at a petting zoo. I was stared at and poked at and whispered about. The blond hair seemed to get them going most of all. (The whole time I was in Saudi Arabia, people offered us ridiculous amounts of money for a few locks of my hair.)

I was completely freaked by the attention, but I understand it now. This was a place where women were shrouded, and treated like second-class citizens, and here I was parading around the airfield, looking to all the locals like a little boy. I was petrified, but I must have seemed brazenly confident, especially for a girl. It's no wonder they didn't know what to make of me; before long, I'd have no idea what to make of myself.

Now, I want to state for the record that I absolutely loved Saudi Arabia. Yes, there were some cultural adjustments I had to deal with, but it was a wonderful thing, to be lifted from my ordinary existence in the suburbs of New York and transported to this exotic place, in the middle of the desert. It was a gift, to be able to grow up amidst such dramatic contrasts. Plus, the compound where we lived was a fun place to grow up: There was a swimming pool, and big open deserts that ran into dunes, and all kinds of things for kids to do. The troubles that found me as an adolescent had nothing to do with my change in environment, and everything to do with my situation at home, as I'll explain.

Despite these feelings of dislocation, I made friends right away. Everyone did, in such a small community. It was about this time that I began to play sports: swimming, touch football, basketball, track, volleyball. I was turning out to be a good athlete—strong, and built for anything. The weight problem my parents had been so worried about was manifesting itself in brawn and muscle and determination. I was bigger than the other kids, the girls especially, but there wasn't a measurable ounce of fat on me. But that wasn't the way Bill saw it.

While we'd hoped that the change of locale would somehow change him, Bill only became more obsessed with weight once we moved to Dhahran. The most galling piece of his obsession was that he started to subject my mother and me to it as well. He couldn't do anything about his own weight, so he set about controlling ours.

My mother had her own insecurities about her size (when I was about nine or ten she showed me pictures of herself at a young age and said she weighed around one hundred sixty and hated the way she felt), so she welcomed the team approach, but I didn't want any part of it. Bill forced us to weigh ourselves regularly, sometimes daily. He watched over what we ate with almost absurd vigilance. It was as if he was on a one-man mission to rid the world of fat, starting at home. At first, his hold over me in this area was subtle, but it began to influence my every waking moment. My entire relationship with Bill, and eventually with my mother, came to be about food and weight. It defined me. It defined us. It became a competition. It was all that mattered. My parents tried every fad diet on the scene: Weight Watchers, egg and grapefruit, all protein/no carbohydrates. Bill kept charts on the wall, tracking our weight.

It was horrible, but I had no idea there was another way to be. Oh, I knew from my friends that there were ways of dealing with food that seemed to be a whole lot less suffocating, it's just that I didn't know there was another way for *us* to be at home. This was the way things had always been in my family, the way they would always be. All around me, kids were eating candy and ice cream, and I could never understand when I went to their houses why they didn't eat all of it at one time. I was already infected with a binge, get-it-while-you-can mentality, crystallized in that moment at Carvel on the way to JFK.

Soon even our vacations had to do with Bill's eating. The entire family traveled with him to Duke University (all the way to North Carolina!) for a special weight-loss program. Think about it: a junior-high-school band instructor, on a mid-level oil company salary, dragging his wife and three children halfway around the world just so we could spend two glorious weeks getting his weight under control. We all stayed in an apartment facility for diet patients and their families. While Bill was off at his workshops and physical examinations, we were left to visit the local mall. Some vacation.

I realize now that this was my introduction to calculated weight loss. At home, I was taught to keep the weight off (or else!), but I was never really told how. At Duke, I began to learn new methods, though what I picked up wasn't exactly the most constructive advice in the world. The common wisdom at the time recommended strict calorie counting, substituting saccharine for sugar, butter buds for butter, diet salad dressing for the real thing. After our "vacation" at Duke, this became a way of life for us. What an awful regimen for a little girl! I was introduced to this so early on, it all seemed very normal.

But how many kids weigh their food before they eat it? What kid chooses Tab over Coke? But that was me. I couldn't think about eating without thinking also of the price of my eating.

I wasn't taught to think of food as fuel, as something I needed to keep my body going. In our house, food was gratification, a guilty pleasure, something to be taken in only under fear of reprisal. We didn't eat to live, we lived to eat. There's an unhealthy difference. It didn't matter that I needed to replenish the calories I'd burned running around all day in the hot sun. It didn't matter that I was hungry, that I was a big girl with a healthy appetite. What mattered was that we had a tendency to gain weight—that's the message that was burned into me—and we had to watch what we ate or risk my stepfather's wrath when it came time to step on the scale.

Now, I'm not sure that the Duke program offered any measurable benefit to Bill, but I think he took a few ideas back home with him, one of which provided the basis for the most clarifying moment of my young life. One afternoon, Bill took out a black marker and told me he wanted to show me something. Then he started highlighting what he perceived to be the potential fat areas on my body. He didn't fully explain what he was doing, or where he got the idea; he just collected me in his arms, mumbled something about helping me to see my "trouble spots" and started drawing on my skin.

I was about twelve. I was tall and big, but I was in no way overweight. I was, however, beginning to feel self-conscious about my appearance, probably because of all the negative reinforcement I was getting at home. Moments like these were no help. Bill offered a vague explanation of how he wanted to show me some of the areas on my body I needed to concentrate on, places I should start to worry about, places that were already a concern to him and my mother. It was for my own good, he said.

I was in my underwear. My stepfather drew circles around my outer thighs, my hips, my arms. When he got to my stomach, I froze. I've since learned, from studying massage therapy, that the stomach is a person's center, probably one of the most sensitive and intimate parts of the body. It's not a sexual thing so much as it is a personal one. Most licensed massage therapists and reflexologists will work your legs, your arms, your back, without a thought, but they'll usually ask for permission before working your stomach. In some states, they're required to ask. Often, clients refuse; they're just too embarrassed to let a stranger so close. Bill certainly didn't ask, and I remember thinking there was something not right about being touched in such a personal way. It was a complete invasion of my privacy and I just checked out. I stood there thinking, *Go ahead, show me what you have to show me, but I'm gone.* And I was.

When he was through, I was crying. I scrambled to the bathroom and tried to scrub the lines from my body, but the stuff wouldn't come off. I was in there for a long time. It's weird, but I don't have any recollection of where my mother was at that specific moment. Was she in the house? Did she even know what was going on? I blamed her as much as I blamed Bill, because she wasn't there to stand up for me. If she was there, she had to have known, but we never talked about it, not at the time, not ever. I felt so incredibly alone in that bathroom—violated and humiliated—and I wanted nothing more than to lose myself in one of my mother's great, warm hugs.

But I was on my own on this one and when I finally thought I'd scrubbed most of the lines off, I put on my bathing suit. I needed to get outside, to put the incident out of my head. It was a bright, hot day, and all the kids were out at the pool, but when I got there one of the boys started pointing at me and laughing. Soon everyone was pointing and laughing. I had no idea what was so funny so I laughed along, but then I looked down and saw the marking in the harsh sunlight.

I raced back home and burst into tears.

I've never lost that moment, and pray I never will, because it is only in the harnessing of such moments that we are able to grow, and move on. I believe that we have to build on our painful childhood memories, to dig into them and learn from them, or we'll just stagnate. Clearly, Bill had no idea what kind of damage he was doing with his black marker. I'm certain he thought he was helping me. And I'm fairly certain that in some ways what he was doing was helpful to him. So for me to sit here, from a healthier perspective, and castigate this man for his insensitivity seems beside the point.

The real point is that it happened. There's no changing that. Even if this specific incident hadn't happened, Bill's negative view of my body would have come through loud and clear. This was just one incident of many underlying that negative view, yet this is the one that stays with me as a kind of touchstone, a marked contrast between the way I lived then versus the way I'm trying to live now. The incident was emblematic of that negative attitude Bill was putting out, just as the Carvel ice cream binge was emblematic of his attitude toward food. Both of these attitudes, I'm sorry to say, are ones I gradually absorbed and internalized to the point where I didn't need Bill around to have them expressed. I felt them too keenly and genuinely myself.

P a u s e

This was what it was like for me, but we all have our own stories, our own watershed moments, our turning points. Think back to your own youth, to the time when you started receiving those first messages that you were not okay, that your shape was not right, that things would be so much better for you if you only were X pounds thinner. I believe there's a dividing line for each of us, a specific moment when we trade our positive or perhaps neutral self-image for a negative one. For me, it coincided with the arrival of my stepfather. For you, it might have been the first time you were teased at school, or an unkind or well-intentioned comment from a complete stranger.

The object here is not to fix blame, but to pinpoint the precise moment when you began to feel less than wonderful because you were made to realize there was more of you than perhaps there should have been. That's all. It's a simple process, but a necessary one. We need to rediscover that moment, reclaim it and turn it around. How did it make you feel? What did it do to the way you approached each day? In what ways did it change the picture of yourself you carried around in your head, or the image that looked back at you in the mirror? How did it affect your attitude toward eating?

Think back to a time before anyone ever expressed any negative opinion about your body. Did you enjoy an idyllic period of almost pure joy, as I did in my early childhood living alone with my mother? If you're lucky, you can recall a time when you felt truly accepted for yourself, exactly as you were. Find that time and relish it. Focus on how you saw yourself then. Walk about in your old shoes and see if they still fit.

In a perfect world none of us would be defined by the way we look, but this is not a perfect world and we'll have to make the best of it. Weight and body-image issues *are* important, but they are not everything. What counts is the way we see ourselves, the way we feel, the way we present ourselves when we make our rounds. Too often, we measure our unhappiness by the number of pounds that separate us from some slender ideal—an ideal that may not be at all appropriate for our body type. This is a key point. We are all born with well-defined skeletal structures (extra-small, small, medium, large, extra-large) and specific body types (ectomorphic, mesomorphic and endormorphic). It is within these permutations and combinations that we find our adult frame. And, once found, there is no changing it: A big-boned person will never become small-boned; an angular ectomorph will never build mass as easily as a muscular mesomorph, and so on.

For those needing a quick definition, a person with an ectomorphic body is naturally tall and angular. An ectomorph has a hard time gaining weight or building and maintaining muscle mass. Ectomorphs tend to be on the thin side; some are diminutive, all appear to be more bones than meat. Think of Shelley Duvall or Don Knotts or the gangly teenager down the block. Most elite long-distance runners are small-boned ectomorphs; some professional basketball players, like Shawn Bradley of the New Jersey Nets, are big-boned ectomorphs.

And clearly, top supermodels like Nadja Auermann appear to be ectomorphic. I stress that they only "appear" to fit this mold, because a lot of models I know go through so much hell trying to stay super-thin, when indeed they are a different body type. I see it all the time. When these women get out of modeling and allow themselves to relax about their weight, all of a sudden another fifteen to twenty pounds pop right on their bodies because they've been needing it. Almost overnight, they resort to their mesomorphic frame, and the extra weight looks right on them.

A mesomorph is someone who is inherently more muscular, with a tendency to gain weight and mass far more easily than an ectomorph. Madonna is a great example of a medium-boned mesomorph. She's definitely a woman with a little mass to her. She can achieve incredible definition in her muscles, but her body doesn't bulk up to where it might be excessive. Or, if it does, she's able to work it off and keep it off. A lot of Broadway dancers are the same way: able to build mass and strength into their frames, without beefing up in weight. Gabrielle Reese, the athlete-model, is mesomorphic. Boxers, power-lifters and bodybuilders usually fit the mold in the extreme. I fit in somewhere in the middle: I gain weight and fatty tissue quickly if I'm not in balance, but if I keep active and nourish myself properly I can maintain my weight at a constant level.

Endomorphs tilt the scales at the other end of

the spectrum. They gain weight and fatty tissue fairly easily, especially if they don't exercise regularly. John Candy was an endomorph who couldn't get his weight under control. Roseanne is an endomorph who has had some success taking the weight off, but she has had to work at it. The defensive linemen on your favorite football team are all proudly endomorphic. Even Marilyn Monroe had endomorphic tendencies. Most people don't remember that about her. She was a size sixteen at the height of her fame, with rounded, curvy hips and a fleshy bottom, and she struggled with her weight her whole life. Being an endomorph does not mean that the muscle mass critical for raising metabolism is unattainable—it is! It just takes an endomorph an extra effort to achieve it.

What this means, for me, is that no diet or exercise program will ever transform me from a mesomorph with slight endomorphic tendencies into a frail, ectomorphic model for Guess? jeans. I am what I am, and I always will be. I can gain weight and fatty tissue pretty easily, but I can also go to a gym and turn myself into a real hard body. What I can't do is will or starve myself into a pair of size-six pants. I will always be about a size fourteen to sixteen. I can't change what I can't change.

Now, it's one thing to understand this concept in the abstract, and quite another to accept it on a personal level. I came to it late. As a teenager in Saudi Arabia, I used to envy my friends. There was something effortless about the way they carried themselves, something natural. They seemed not to worry about their appearance: they just . . . appeared. I couldn't imagine that these girls ever worried about what to eat, or what to wear, or what to say. But I worried constantly. Coming from my house, where I was judged by how much I weighed and criticized for the slightest transgression, the idea of moving about with true confidence was too good to be believed. I walked around with a huge smile on my face, radiating what I hoped was confidence, but on the inside I was incredibly insecure and unsure of myself. I was trying to fool myself along with the rest of the world.

It was an agonizing lesson, when I finally got it, but one we all have to process at one time or another. It's a lesson I take with me when I lecture to school groups around the country. I tell kids that the only way to make your body the best it can be is to understand it, and to work within your body-type parameters. Know what's possible and what's impossible. Know where to begin, and what to expect.

Think of yourself like a balloon, I say. They come in all shapes and sizes—classic round balloons, oval balloons, snake-skinny party animal balloons. No amount of hot air can blow a skinny balloon into a round one; put in too much air and the balloon will pop. And yet if you don't put in enough, the balloon will appear listless; it won't achieve its intended shape.

I'm not suggesting we accept ourselves exactly as we are, carte blanche. True beauty is not monolithic. It is inclusive and appreciative of variety and balance. I simply refuse to put the emphasis on pounds or size. We live in a society that puts weight and shape in purely cosmetic terms, but I try to think of my body in terms of health. I don't count calories, but I do make sure I consume the right mix of vitamins and nutrients to get my body the fuel it requires. I look at what I eat in terms of how it might make me feel as the day goes along.

I can understand how my parents might have been alarmed by my size, but many children are just larger than their peers. What I can't accept is the way they responded to that alarm. There's no good reason to teach a child to think less of herself simply because she casts a bigger shadow than the other kids her age. When I have children, there'll be a moratorium on the word *fat* in our house. It simply won't be a part of our day-to-day, no matter what we all look like. For us, the emphasis will be on health. I'll work hard to keep my child's head free of the notion that her size has anything to do with her attitude, to encourage her to be how she wants and what she wants no matter what.

What body type are you? Ectomorph? Mesomorph? Endomorph? Maybe somewhere in between? If you happen to be a mesomorph with endomorphic propensities or if you're a true endomorph, this doesn't mean that you have to be obese. What it does mean, most likely, is that you are large—like me!—certainly larger than the commonly accepted ideal.

I encourage you to reject this "ideal." It's not a body image you should be aiming for. If you had strawberry-blond hair and freckles you'd know it would be ludicrous to aim for exotic Asian good looks. Well, it's just as ludicrous for women with our body type to hanker after a type that by definition is not to be ours. So figure out what your body type is and then aim for the appropriate ideal if you want to aim for anything. You can start by asking yourself some questions:

Is my body serving me well? Am I doing what

I can to make the most of what I have? How do I *feel?* Am I energetic? Does my body aid me in accomplishing all I hope to accomplish? Or does it get in the way, leaving me tired and drained if I try to do too much?

The real key here for starters is knowing and accepting your body type. Only then can you begin to get yourself back to that frame of mind you had as a kid, when you accepted yourself as you were—probably without thinking about it.

3

*L*eaving *H*ome

I was in no way prepared for what happened next. The doctors at the Aramco compound found a spot on my mother's lung during a routine examination. (We all had to take annual tuberculosis X rays while we were there.) By the time they caught it, Mom's cancer had spread to the extent that there was little hope.

This news was devastating. My mother was only thirty-eight; I was fifteen. There's not a teenage girl alive who doesn't need her mother, but I felt I needed mine more than most. I couldn't imagine a life without her. I'd be completely lost, and alone.

I had a strangely comforting dream the night before I was told my mother was sick. More than anything else, that's what got me through. I never had a dream like it, before or since. I was staying overnight at a friend's house and I dreamed I saw heaven. It was all very ethereal and hazy, but what registered was that I was in the presence of tremendous love and understanding. I was a visitor, and not meant to stay, but I felt calm and safe and strong. I remember not wanting to leave, but being told that it was not my time. It was a very spiritual dream, and though I woke in the middle of the night I wasn't scared or confused. The dream itself might have been fuzzy, but what it had to tell me became so amazingly clear. The more I thought about it, the stronger I felt, and the more deeply I believed that this strength would be for a purpose. When my mother told me her news the next day, I took it far more calmly than I could have before.

Bill decided to transfer to the oil company's affiliate offices in Houston so Mom could be in a city where she'd get the finest medical attention, and my family settled in for the ordeal ahead. I'd already applied to several American prep schools (there was no high school at the Aramco compound), so we'd long planned for me to attend a boarding school back in the States.

I couldn't leave home now, I thought, not with my mother as sick as she was, not with Bill's already thin patience being spread even thinner, not with a brother and new baby sister unable to help themselves. But my mother was adamant: She knew how much I'd been looking forward to going away and she was determined that her illness affect her children's lives as little as possible. Of course there was no way she could buffer us ultimately, but she would try to for as long as she could. So at my mother's insistence, and frankly with some relief, I went off to the Kent School in Kent, Connecticut.

Going away to school was even more liberating than I thought it would be. I was on my own in a totally new environment. Best of all, I was out from under Bill's rules, and that's what stood out. Eating had always been the focus of so much anxiety and so many rules in our house, I wasn't prepared for the casual abundance of meals in the dining hall. We ate boarding-house style, with huge platters set out in front of us. At home, we rarely strayed from Mom's Weight Watchers cookbook. Everything was healthy and portions were carefully measured. At Kent, there were wonderful mounds of potatoes, platters filled with meats and cheeses, bottomless dessert trays. The contrast was startling.

I might have approached each meal like one of

those last-chance sundaes at the JFK Carvel. But I
didn't. Although there wasn't anyone standing by my
plate weighing my food and restraining me from eating any more than a predetermined amount, I quickly
picked up on the attitudes expressed about eating by
the other girls in my class. I'd hear them talking:
"Oh, I'm not gonna have anything tonight." "I have
to lose a few pounds." "I'm visiting my boyfriend this
weekend, so I'll just drink some juice." Juice? With
all that good stuff around? What was wrong with
these people? I couldn't understand it. But after a few
weeks of seeing these girls control themselves, I felt
uncomfortable reaching for the generous helpings I
craved. This is where I believe my personal relationship with food began to change. Actually, to put a
finer point on it, it's where my relationship with
food truly began. I was on my own, developing eating habits that revolved around how my jeans fit
(when we were out of our uniforms), the emotional
eating around going home for a vacation, whether I
was winning or losing, feeling lonely or depressed.
Food was something more than fuel for me, and at
the same time something less. I went from periods
of overeating to periods of eating with "such self-
control," and the only constant was my uncertainty.
For the most part, I ate what I wanted, and then
some. I deserved it, right? I used to have a tape play

in my head when I tried to restrain myself. "It's here for me to eat and no one is telling me to stop." "It tastes so good, I'll have just a bit more." Each time I "indulged," I found myself back in my dorm room with another tape playing in my head that tore me down for letting myself be so weak. There were times I avoided food altogether to show myself I could do it . . . to be good. But I always became so famished the cycle would repeat itself over and over. During this time, I had no clue how to eat. I didn't have it in me to eat until I was full, to sit back and enjoy what I had just eaten. All I knew was I wanted more.

I know now that even people who weren't raised under the obsessive influences of someone like my stepfather tend to flipflop badly when first charged with feeding themselves, or monitoring their own eating habits. That's a big responsibility, and I must confess I didn't handle it all that well. At school, we had family-style eating, which meant platters of food were placed on each table in the dining hall with an unlimited supply of more in the kitchen. A lot of the foods we ate were new to me and not usually served at home, so I was breaking away from the rigidity I was used to. Another aspect of the dining room is that we changed seating assignments regularly, so I got to see how other people ate. A garden variety. Some girls ate like me, and it made me feel good that

I wasn't the only one with the "healthy appetite." When I think back about it, I probably was as hungry as I was because physically I was working out for one team or another. The guilt was something else entirely. It was an emotional connection that led me away from appreciating my size for what it was, or my appetite for what it meant. I was on this cycle to starve myself down to what some of my friends saw as the perfect figure, never realizing that it wasn't anywhere near the perfect figure for me.

I couldn't see that. What I could see were pounds lost or gained equaling success or failure. All I could see was that I wasn't like the other girls who didn't have a problem passing up their servings because they were "not hungry." They had all the answers. What restraint! They seemed to carry such confidence against food, something that I tried and tried to do but kept failing at. Before long, though, I saw that they lost weight and bragged about how they did it. The compliments would just pour. I found if I lost weight, I too got compliments, and I liked that. So food was to be used for compliments as well. All the time I kept thinking, if the other kids can do it, so can I. Desserts looked scrumptious, but I valued myself in terms of my ability to resist them. To refuse a cake or a portion of dinner was victory, but then I'd go back to my room and scream. No matter how much I tried to control myself at the meals, I ate either very little or too much. Back and forth, round and round. Most nights, I ended up in my dorm room praising my self-restraint or beating myself up for giving in. This was so routine that it became the only way I dealt with food for a very long time.

The crazy part is that no matter how much I denied myself at meals, I'd step on a friend's scale in the dorm or at the gym only to find out I hadn't even lost an ounce. Not a single ounce! Now I was certain that there was something wrong with me. My approach to food was fine: I ate very little on days following the nights I overate. Plain and simple. My body was letting me down. But I wasn't being completely honest with myself. I wouldn't eat "a lot" for a week in the dining hall, but I'd be so famished at night in my room that no amount of Doritos, peanut M&Ms, or order-in pizza could satisfy me. I began to yo-yo between two weight points. I'd put on six or seven pounds (mostly through late-night snacking) and then starve myself back to my baseline weight—about one hundred sixty pounds. I was almost full height, a size twelve, but I was conditioned to think of myself as a young girl with a weight problem. Talk about the devastation when I stepped off the scale once I saw I gained weight. I can remember my heart rate go up, a sick feeling in the pit of my stomach, and then the tape would start playing again: "You're no good." "You can't even stay a consistent weight." "What's wrong with you?" "If you don't watch it you're going to end up fat!" If only I weighed one hundred fifty-five! Just five pounds less! It would make all the difference. It's tough to erase an image you've held for your entire life, even if you know it to be false.

The other girls seemed to have no trouble maintaining their figures, but I was all over the place. I just couldn't get a handle on it. My self-confidence and self-esteem were as unsteady as my eating patterns. One minute I'd been feeling, *I'm the best.* Then, it would be, *I'm not good enough. I can handle it; I don't know what I'm doing. I'm thin; I'm fat. Everything will be okay; nothing will be right again.* Some guy would check me out in class and my self-esteem would soar, but then I'd pass a mirror or step on a scale and ride it right back down again. (That's another thing: Even *without* the pressure of Bill's weigh-ins, he had me so conditioned that I policed myself on his behalf.)

I found myself trying very, very hard to lose weight, and then not worrying about it. One day, it was the most important thing in the world, and the next it could not have mattered less. Eating began to have nothing to do with fueling my body and everything to do with punishing or rewarding myself. I had never been like this before. I ate because I felt guilty, not because I was hungry. I starved myself because the other girls were doing it. I ate because I was lonely. I starved myself because I didn't deserve to eat. I ate because I felt good about myself, or because I felt rotten. Worst of all, I was making inappropriate connections between food and rewards and punishments, connections it would take me a long time to break.

I was a compulsive eater. I didn't know it at the time, but I was a textbook case, and the most peculiar thing was that it seemed to come out of nowhere. Sure, I had been focused on my weight since my mother remarried, and yes, I was somewhat larger than most of my peers, but I think it was the contradiction between our approach to food under my parents' roof and the casual way it was dealt with now that I was out on my own that had me so flustered.

Clearly, my mother's illness contributed to my confusion—about food and everything else. I was away from home at a time I felt I should have been near. Perhaps the change in weather also had something to do with my change in appetite. I'd spent the past seven years in the desert, and the previous summer in Houston, so the chill of New England naturally took some getting used to. Granted, there's no widely accepted physiological correlation between diet and weather, but it makes sense. If someone had clued me in to the *possibility* that my body needed another layer of fat or insulation to handle the colder temperatures, even if it was just an old wives' tale, my unpredictable eating habits would have been easier to understand.

At sixteen years old, I couldn't see food as necessary fuel. In our house, there were only good foods and bad foods. There were good amounts and bad amounts. I judged what I ate in black and white; there was no gray. Like most girls, I went away to school fretting about the Freshman Ten—the extra ten pounds or so that many students are likely to gain their first year away from home. My parents cautioned me about it, but their warnings were no match for the variety of foods (good *and* bad), and the freedom to eat whatever I wanted, whenever I wanted.

Meanwhile, whenever I went back home, my parents' focus remained on my weight. Despite everything else going on—my studies, my mother's health—it kept coming back to that. Even while I was at school, my parents would get the message through. Bill usually signed his letters, "How's your weight? Love, Dad." (I've kept them, all these years, to remind myself how things were.) Phone calls, too.

And my stepfather and Mom were always a little too quick to ask about my diet.

My emotional eating disorder—and that's what it was!—was far more benign than most, but at the time it felt bigger than I could handle on my own. Now that I've gotten past it, I'm still working to find the link between the way I am today and the way I was as a girl. It wasn't *just* about eating for me, I realize now. Clearly, my relationships with other people were connected to my various relationships with food.

All around me, as I grew up and moved on, I saw other people connecting in ways I could not. (I'm getting ahead of my story a little bit, so bear with me here.) I didn't get how to interact with people in a mature relationship. I had a lot of good, casual friends, but only one really close friend. When I started to date, I dated mostly strong, domineering guys, who were a lot more like my stepfather than I would have ever considered at the time. It was an unhealthy way to be, and I don't mean simply in terms of the negative body image I carried with me from my time at home. It was more than that. Whenever I felt lost, or bottomless, or only loosely connected to my present situation, I handled things the way I had handled them as a child. I shut my eyes against the world, agreed, and went along.

More and more, I found myself not being able to

get close to other people. I wanted intimacy, but I didn't know how to find it, or where to look. I certainly couldn't find it at home. This wanting infected everything, and I couldn't figure it out. I spent a lot of time alone. When I thought about it, I imagined the distance I put between myself and others had something to do with the way my mother always left the house with a smile on her face, no matter what sadness or uncertainty she carried in her heart. Like a child, I admired that, without appreciating the cost. She always *seemed* happy, even when she wasn't.

When I thought about it some more, I understood that this walking about without expressing a true emotion was a learned behavior, to keep from rocking the boat, and if I could learn it I could just as well unlearn it. I took a pragmatic view, and began to filter my present-day experiences against what I remembered from childhood. At first, I felt as if I could cry forever and ever. Underneath all my protective layers, I was still this untethered child, but now I had finally reached a place of security that allowed me to explore what had for so long been hidden.

Back at Kent, away from home for the first time, I was trying to find a way to deal with boyfriends and dating, which was a whole other muddle. There I was, on a coed campus, at a time when most of my girlfriends were starting to see themselves from their boyfriends' perspectives. I was hopelessly confused. I had enough trouble getting (and keeping) a positive image of myself in my own head, without worrying about having it filtered through some guy. But I went through the motions, like everyone else.

My first honest-to-goodness kiss had been down in North Carolina, on our diet vacation at Duke, and even this moment was tinged with uncertainty. We were in a car, and the kiss itself was actually quite nice—not too long, not too short—but it wasn't until he walked me to the door that I realized this boy had probably planned his move pretty carefully. I was about six or seven inches taller than he was, and there was no way he could have kissed me with any kind of style unless we were both sitting down. When he walked me to the door, he didn't even attempt a good-night kiss, which in my head I took to mean I was way too tall to be worth the trouble.

Things weren't any better in high school. I was much more mature physically than most of the boys on campus. I was built. But I couldn't help thinking there was something wrong with me, something I could change. The boys I liked seemed to always go for someone about a foot shorter, and far more petite. And the boys who did show an interest were always navigating their way into more comfortable kissing positions. It would have been funny if I wasn't the one stuck at the other end. For a while at Kent, I dated this one guy who put my car-kissing friend at Duke to shame. He was embarrassed when I leaned down to kiss him, so he constantly placed us in situations more to his advantage. He'd sit on a fence and have me lean into him, or he'd turn to me on the slope of a hill. As I recall, we did a lot of our necking sitting down. We never really talked about it, but his efforts were transparent, and I was torn between thinking there was something sweet about him and thinking there was something pathetic about me.

Really, to have to factor this other piece into what was already a pretty trying equation was more than most teenagers could have handled, and I didn't do such a good job of it. No wonder I sometimes ate to console myself. What I needed was some heavy-duty positive reinforcement, something to get me feeling good about myself again.

*P*ause

Matters of the heart remain uneasy ground for most people. Self-confidence flags. People wonder if they're attractive enough, smart enough, witty enough. From talking to friends I know that dating—for lack of a better word—is a trying experience even for those who by rights seem to have no reason to feel anxious: the beautiful, the intelligent, the svelte.

For women, size remains an issue when it comes to dating and sex. For me, my size has been a fact I've had to contend with from my first kiss on. It's a fact of my life: I was bigger than nearly every guy I ever dated. I'm bigger than my husband now.

I think it's important to acknowledge that size may remain a sensitive point for you when it comes to intimacy. I know that when I was in college and in a rather intimate moment with a new boyfriend, he made an offhand comment about being afraid I would squash him. Even though I know he meant it as something of a joke, his remark stayed with me long after we broke up. I'd often wonder how many other guys were secretly worried about the very same thing, but were too polite, too shy or too sensitive themselves to say anything.

I'd be less than honest if I said this crack didn't bother me. It did. The point is, I didn't let it defeat me. I refused to dwell on it or brood over it. And I reminded myself what I knew from talking to friends: All of us worry about our deficiencies—real or imagined—particularly when it comes to dating. Being big just happens to be my personal point of concern. I have friends for whom size isn't an issue, but who are bothered by equally troubling worries instead. I have one good friend who is pretty flat-chested. She's always secretly worried about what a turn-off her lack of a feminine figure will be, particularly without clothes. At the very moment she is about to be most intimate, she feels the least confident. A wave of panic comes over her and she has to remind herself to take a deep, calming breath. Another friend is anxious about her thick thighs. Someone else may be bothered by being too short or too thin.

My point is, everybody's got something about themselves that troubles them when it comes to physical intimacy. For you it may be your size. If it is, you might try to remind yourself that if it weren't this, it could be something else. And you could also remind yourself that if you are becoming more intimate with a guy, it's not as if your size can come as a surprise to him! You might also consider that your size—your curves and womanly figure—might be part of your attraction. Many men prefer more shapely women even if that isn't the trendy body type put forth in the media.

I don't recommend denial as a tactic in dealing with your size when it comes to relationships and intimacy. It's up to you how to handle it beyond that. For some, it may be easier to leave any difference in size as something tacitly understood, the way my very first date left it. He subtly orchestrated our more romantic moments so that size wasn't an issue; we only kissed while sitting, never standing up. For others, a more direct approach may be in order. In these cases, humor always helps. And sometimes you may make your date more comfortable by defusing the issue first.

You'll probably find that one approach works well in one instance while a different situation or a different guy suggests a different approach. And in every situation, you need to decide what works for you. So think about being flexible. Think about trying to change tactics. And remember: Being bigger than the preferred "ideal" doesn't make you uniquely susceptible to pangs of low self-esteem and self-doubt. From talking to others I know that while the particulars may vary from person to person, those negative feelings are resoundingly the same. So the real issue is contending with the low self-esteem and self-doubt. Our size is just the source of insecurity our negative selves may use to erode our confidence. Don't let it happen! When your negative self talks to you, talk back!

"It's not what happens to you that matters," Rose Kennedy once said. "It's how you handle it." Taking a cue from her, I'd say it's not your size that matters, it's how you handle it. Attitude is key. And attitude isn't something determined from birth, like eye color. Attitude is definitely something you can work on, develop and shape. Shape it to serve your happiness.

4

Finding Myself

I didn't know it at the time, but I lacked a focus for my energies. I needed something to distract me from my terrors of my mother's illness, the uncertainties of the Kent dining hall, and the awkwardness of adolescence, but I also needed to ground myself in some sort of routine. I needed a challenge.

I found it accidentally on the girls' crew team. My first year away at school I actually went out for basketball. I loved playing hoops, but I seemed to be so much better at it than the other girls that there was no challenge in it, no reward. I don't mean to boast, but I want to set the scene for what happened next.

I left basketball tryouts feeling a bit disillusioned about the season ahead; the level of competition was not what I expected, and I was moping around figuring what to do about it when I came upon a group of girls rowing in longboats across the pond. The crew team rowed on the nearby Housatonic River, but the pond was good enough for tryouts. I thought, What an odd-looking sport! I'd never seen such a thing. As a matter of fact, I don't think I'd ever even been in a boat. I stood looking on for the longest time, until the coach walked over and started checking *me* out. He looked me over from head to toe. Finally he said, "I think you'll be great."

Me? Great? At what?

Coach must have recognized the look of confusion on my face for what it was, because he answered my questions before I could get them out. "You're tall," he explained. "And you've got muscles. Let's just get you in a boat and see what happens."

What happened was I tipped over. He'd put me in a one-person boat, and those singles tend to tip pretty easily, but once I righted myself and figured out what to do, it turned out that I had a nice, long stroke. There was a grace and power about rowing that I could never have imagined. That first day, I was hooked, and I signed on to the team right there.

We rowed in eight-person boats. I loved being

part of a team. It gave me that sense of all of us being in it together. I also loved the fact that we were all tall, and stocky. For crew, mine was the preferred body type. And I loved the camaraderie. I loved that I was not alone.

Right away, rowing helped me to see that my body could really, really work for me. My body actually made the boat move! I felt each good stroke through every muscle—legs, back, arms—and I left each practice knowing I had pushed myself hard and well.

I had always been athletic, and now that I was exercising these muscles in an organized way I began to look at myself in a different manner. I no longer pined for a body I could never have, or determined to shape myself to meet the expectations of others; I was all for putting what I *did* have to optimum use and dedicating myself to my new purpose.

Without a doubt, crew effected the most positive change in my life up to that point. Whereas before my body had seemed to me like an enemy, ever thwarting my plans and desires, now my body was my friend: a source of pride and strength, full of power valued by my teammate friends.

The more I trained, the harder my body got. I was still big—if anything, my shoulders and the muscles in my arms, legs and back became even more developed. But my muscles were toned. I felt so strong and with that strength came a special confidence. I didn't need to worry so much about what I ate any more. My body was an engine requiring plenty of fuel. With high calorie-burning training sessions sometimes as frequently as twice a day, this was the first time in my life that it seemed I really could eat anything and not suffer the effects. I was immune! I could eat with impunity.

For the first time, I had a goal that was bigger than myself. I belonged. I was part of a team. My focus wasn't on keeping my weight down; as a matter of fact, my coach wanted me to bulk up a bit, to improve my strength and stamina. I learned to appreciate my body by seeing it through the eyes of my coach and my teammates, and by seeing what it could do when I put it to the test.

Crew was a critical watershed for me in two significant ways. For one thing, through crew I was first able to appreciate some of the strengths associated with my size—the concept of size as an asset was totally new to me. Second, crew provided me with a true wellspring of self-esteem. My success in the sport left me feeling good about myself due to tangible achievements unrelated to how I was feeling about my body. For a number of reasons it was the perfect endeavor for me at that time.

Before crew, being big and the struggle to be slim

occupied my thoughts. With crew, training came to occupy not only my thoughts but my entire life.

Crew is an obsessive sport. For me, the obsessiveness was part of the attraction. Not only did it give me self-esteem and the sense of controlling my body, it also let me focus on the sport to the exclusion of other issues in my life—issues I wasn't prepared or inclined to deal with. Of course, I only see this in retrospect. I didn't fully appreciate it at the time. And while others may feel I used crew in a bad way to obscure these other issues, I also believe it is crew that got me through.

My mother's cancer is the toughest thing I've ever had to deal with. It felt especially tough then.

Although I looked big, in my high-school years, I already felt fragile between the kinds of anxieties and insecurities any teen feels and the particular issues I faced being bigger than my peers and the legacy of Bill's peculiar mind-set about weight. Dealing with a parent's terminal illness is never easy, but given everything else I was experiencing emotionally, I felt distinctly ill-equipped to deal with it then. I felt guilty about not being with my mother even though I knew I was where she wanted me to be. She was insistent that her illness not disrupt my life any more than it had to. But I still felt very uneasy about not being by her side even as I complied with her wishes.

Compounding my sense of guilt was the fact that as much as I wanted to be with my mother, I really did enjoy being away at school. And it was such a relief to be away from Bill!

The more I threw myself into crew, the more I forgot those anxieties. For most of my waking hours, I was either training hard or recovering from all that training. Rowing is exhausting. I was often literally too tired to worry about too much. Then there were the endorphins.

Endorphins are our body's natural uppers. They are secreted after periods of sustained physical exertion. Endorphins are what cause the famed "runner's high" experienced by distance runners and even joggers. There's no doubt about it: Aerobic exercise stimulates an ebullience, a real upswing in mood. That's why exercise can often provide a drug-free way of dealing with stress.

Endorphins definitely helped me get through a lot of my tough days in high school. I would never wish my crew days away. At the same time, I now believe that endorphins helped to mask a lot of what was going on with me at the time. Though they helped me get through a difficult period, they did so by enhancing my capabilities for avoidance. After a hard workout, my spirits would soar, riding the endorphin tide. It's a great way to feel but it doesn't leave you poised for rigorous soul-searching or focusing on more heart-rending issues.

So while I remain a huge booster of exercise and competitive athletics, I also acknowledge their limits. But it was still a few years before I could put exercise in proper perspective.

*P*ause

For me, crew became the foundation for almost everything I've done since. No, it didn't give me the slim, trim figure of my adolescent dreams, but it did help me to develop a honed, well-muscled body, which became a new point of satisfaction and pride. It taught me the benefits of hard work and dedication. And it taught me that no goal was too small if you put your heart and soul into it; the only thing that matters is that it matters to you. In crew, you train months and months to achieve the perfect six minutes out on the water. That's all our races were, six minutes, and yet those six minutes were stretched out in slow motion and charged with all kinds of meaning. Really, those six minutes were everything, and when we were out there, competing, the hard effort we put into it was so totally worth it.

Crew also helped me to feel things much more intensely than I ever had, and to get as much as I possibly could out of every last moment. It made me think, and encouraged me to work through my problems—systematically and diligently. The sport is a constant reminder that good things come with patience and perseverance.

Of course, there was a price to all those life lessons, and to the well-toned muscles that came with the package. The only way to keep up a body like that is through rigorous training several hours a day, every day. That doesn't leave too much room for anything else in your life. I believe there's a time and a place for everything. High school and college are definitely the right time for this obsessive pursuit of excellence through sports. At least it was for me. But as a lifetime strategy it isn't quite so effective, mainly because of the huge drain it puts on your time. At just the period in your life that you need to channel your energies into a career or a lasting relationship, it's not possible to maintain a training regimen involving three to four hours of workouts per day. I was willing to devote myself to crew in my school years. It was appropriate then. But I don't find that that kind of devotion is compatible with my goals and pastimes now. And if I'm not willing to put in the time, I have to be willing to give up the hard body.

It may be appropriate for someone like Demi Moore or Madonna to spend three hours a day with a personal trainer. Their looks are their livelihood. But I'll tell you, even as someone who currently makes her livelihood through her looks, I don't feel there are enough hours in the day to warrant that kind of devotion to the body perfect. Do I exercise? You bet. Only it's likely to be three days a week, not six or seven. As a result, I feel healthy and strong even if I'm no longer muscled enough to be cast as a well-oiled female star opposite a Jean-Claude Van Damme or Arnold Schwarzenegger.

And as far as endorphins go, I still look forward to that amazing sense of well-being that comes after a hard, sweaty session on my bike or in the gym. But there's an appropriateness to the role they play in my life now too. As a result, I feel that I am living my life in a way I didn't always in high school and college. I'm really living it, not just sailing above it.

5

Holding On

Just as I was beginning to feel connected at school, things began to unravel at home. Mom was getting worse. Although I had been deferring to her wishes about remaining in school, even she understood that this was my last chance to be with her. So the visits home became more frequent, and our phone calls stretched on into the night. The weaker Mom became, the stronger I tried to be, but I was only barely holding it together on the surface.

It was excruciating for me to watch my mother waste away. Sometimes the change in her between visits was dramatic, even when the interim was only a matter of weeks. I remember feeling so helpless in the face of my mother's cancer. Intellectually, I guess I understood that there wasn't much anyone could do for her, but emotionally all I knew was that she had always been there for me. She had protected me and encouraged me. I wanted to protect and encourage her.

Being home was problematic for me in other ways. I was so pleased with my tough, crew-honed body, but in Bill's eyes I was only bigger than ever. Even my mother wasn't sure she liked my strong new physique. She wanted her little girl back and said so. I see now that my mother may simply have been nostalgic for an earlier, more carefree time, but I took her literally: I was still too big to be pleasing.

So between the stress of my mother's deteriorating health, my efforts to keep it together, and the disconnect between the positive feedback I was getting from my coach versus my very negative reviews at home, I began to crack. I reverted to some of my old eating patterns in the cafeteria, and in my room at night.

Even though I was still working out at crew, burning major calories, I was still beating myself up for eating so much. I just couldn't find the right balance. I was "bad" one day, and "good" the next, and it got to where I could no longer regulate my appetites. It's clear to me now that my eating habits were out of control, but I think I even knew it then. I think I knew that this was my way of attempting to reconcile my old beliefs about an ideal body image—beliefs that were getting a sudden renewed boost from home—with my fledgling concept of a bigger, more honed, muscular paradigm presented through crew. The result wasn't healthy, physically or emotionally.

By February 1979, Mom couldn't hold on any longer. I flew down to Houston to be at her side, but all I could do was sit with her and hold her hand and tell her that I loved her. It's funny, but I remember these last moments as being between me and my mother. It's as if no one else was there, when I know that Bill was present. But in my mind's eye, it was as if Mom and I were back in our Manhattan apartment, on our own. It was just the two of us—again, at last.

We'd sit up together late into the night, talking and holding hands. We both knew she was dying, and I had it in my head that I should be as brave as I knew my mother to be. I wanted to face the truth. We cried together, but they were good tears, peaceful tears. I told my mother about how I sometimes thought of her dying as a chance for her to chart our next adventure. I thought of where she was going and imagined we would join her someday.

After a while, she'd drift off to sleep, but I'd stay up with her for as long as I could. Her hand in mine was a link to the little girl I was and to the woman I hoped to be. I can still hear my mother's quiet breathing from those late nights together, and I will always treasure those final moments. In them, I felt I knew where my mother was going, that there would be no separating us, that there was more to life than our time on this earth, that we would all be okay.

I still drew strength from that dream I'd had back in Dhahran the night before I learned something was wrong with my mother. I also drew strength from my faith. I believed. And so did Mom. She had always been a religious person. We went to church every Sunday in the States, every Friday in the desert. Mom was in great pain in the end, but she died knowing that she had done the best she could for her family. She was confident she'd be looking out for us from above.

Bill tried to be there for me after Mom died. He really did. He kept coming to me and saying, "We have to talk about this, we have to be open about this, we have to figure this out." I couldn't see what there was to figure, though I appreciated his reaching out to me.

We tried to work our way through my mother's death together, but an uncomfortable silence seemed to follow us around. We couldn't even talk to each other under normal circumstances, so we certainly couldn't communicate then. Looking back on it, I can still see that Bill was doing a lot of grieving on his own, and that my younger brother and sister required a little more attention than I did in the days immediately following my mother's death. So essentially I was left to mourn by myself. This wasn't necessarily so bad, except I didn't do such a good job of it, not for several years. I was so busy trying to be strong that I never really let myself grieve. I went back to school in Connecticut sooner than I should have and tried to put myself back on course too soon. I wasn't ready to do anything, and yet I tried to do it all, alone.

This is where my friends checked back in. They'd invite me home with them on weekends, and their families were great. They made me feel like I belonged, and helped to ease me back into a temporary normality. There was love in my house, but it wasn't expressed the way it was in these homes. Around these dinner tables, together, these parents worked to build their children up, not tear them down. I'd lie awake those nights, in my friends' bedrooms, and against the sounds of their breathing imagine what my life might have been like in a more nourishing environment.

The summer after my mother died, when I was away from Kent and from rowing, I took another turn for the worse. I became paranoid about gaining weight. I starved myself as much as I could. I was afraid to work out because it would make me hungry. I was on the scale constantly. I couldn't sleep at night, I was so afraid of getting fat. If Mom wanted me to be her little girl, then I would be her little girl. I developed a completely unrealistic vision of myself, of what I could be. Every reminder that I was falling short left me depressed and confused.

I've often wondered if my new obsession with my body image was my expression of the mourning process. I'd never mourned my mother's death in the traditional way. There was no funeral. I cried, but every time I did I tried not to. Even through my tears I was trying to hold something back. I couldn't let Bill see me weak and scared. I wanted to be strong for my brother and sister. And I didn't want my friends to know how helpless I was feeling. I guess I had everyone fooled. People would come up to me all the time and ask how I was handling things so well. I never had an answer. It felt like things were handling me.

By the time school rolled around again, I was ready to return to reclaim the pieces of myself that had to do with crew. I rediscovered my drive for the sport but it was a while before I got a grip on my eating problem.

Without meaning to, without even knowing it, I'd developed a real fixation on being thin. It may have had to do with pleasing my mother at first, but it soon took on a life quite its own.

I began obsessing about specific body parts: my hips, my thighs, my butt. Maybe I thought I could better concentrate on one particular area than on the whole package. Even though I knew I had to give my body proper fuel as I continued to train, I resisted. I denied myself the food I needed, and then, in moments of desperation and hunger, I scrambled to take in as many calories as I could. Without meaning to, I was back to the eating cycle I'd gone on during those early days at Kent and again during that winter when my mother got sicker: I ate like a rabbit in front of my friends in the dining hall, then binged on junk food in my room at night. This pattern was unhealthy enough for me as a freshman, but now that I was a varsity athlete, it was disastrous. I was literally making myself sick. My crew performance suffered. I'd feel weak during practice, no doubt in part due to my extraordinarily poor nutrition. My coach wondered what was going on but suspected that I was still suffering from my mother's death.

Really, I was starting to suffer from my *response* to

my mother's death, not her death itself. But it was a while before anyone had a real fix on what was going on with me—including me.

I've often wondered about the masks we wear as we walk through this life, the faces we put on to make ourselves feel better or chase the world away. There was a time when I had enough masks to throw my own Halloween party, and there are still a few kicking around just waiting for the right occasion. Somewhere in me there's a brave face to see me through almost any situation. I inherited it from my mother, and I wore it to best (or worst) effect on her death.

I can still see myself, sitting on my mother's hospital bed, with all of these horrifying tubes coming out of her. She looked grotesque, but I chose not to see it. To me, she was beautiful. She looked like she did when I was a small child. She was my mother. I was her little girl. Nothing bad could ever happen.

When my mother was dying, I wore my mask of denial like a shield, to the point where people must have thought I was in shock. And I was. The only place I had ever felt safe and whole was in my mother's arms, and now that she was about to breathe her last, now that I was about to be left alone in a family I feared had no real place for me, I refused to believe it.

I set this out as a caution: It's one thing to delude

the rest of the world into thinking you're in control, or certain of your place within it, but you cross a line when you delude yourself. I crossed that line with my mother's death, big time. I was simply unable to take a clear view. Those who suffer from eating disorders or struggle with negative body image have trouble accepting their own circumstances, but the problems don't always reach clinical proportions. I've known men and women so totally obsessed with their appearances that they've never been able to see themselves the way they really are. I've known obnoxious people who thought they were charming, and charming people who thought they were obnoxious. I've known people whose self-esteem was so low they had to look up to look down on themselves, and yet they still met each day with the kind of false confidence that almost always leads to disappointment. Every model I've ever worked with has at one time or another lied to a client about her measurements, or put herself up for an assignment for which she was clearly not qualified.

Here's what I think: If we can't see ourselves as we truly are, we can never present ourselves as we wish to be seen. If we can't accept what's happening and address it honestly, we'll never find a way to deal with it in real terms. The masks we hide behind leave us more exposed than protected; what we choose to conceal often tells more about us than what we reveal.

I used to believe that we had two choices, when we stepped outside to meet each new day—we could be happy or we could be sad. It seemed so basic. But now I think we need to sway within the gray a bit, and allow ourselves the whole spectrum of emotions. We can be a little happy, and a little sad, and a little somewhere in between. We can mourn *and* celebrate. We can be confident *and* unsure of ourselves, shy *and* outgoing, trusting *and* cautious.

We can do what we have to do, and be who we are.

*P*ause

Through crew, I was close to resolving the huge gap between my ideal for my body and reality when my mother grew sicker. Crew had been helping me to forge a better, more realistic sense of self and an ideal to aim for that was based on my body type rather than wishful thinking. But I was still off-balance; I hadn't settled permanently in this new view, so Mom's worsening condition was enough to knock me off keel.

Tough times come to nearly everyone at one point or another. If you have an uneasy relationship with eating and your body image to begin with, these same areas may be your most vulnerable when you're under extraordinary stress. If you'd been making progress, a death in the family, a failed romance, a lost job or ill health may send you backsliding to old ways. As you can see, that's what happened to me. Before I knew it I was on my emotional roller-coaster ride of overeating and of denying myself food.

This is why I think it is to important to work hard to develop healthier eating habits, a better relationship with food, and an appropriate image of your body at its best. The more you can develop these patterns, the more you can walk them and live them, the less likely you will be to revert so totally to those bad old ways.

Nobody's perfect and few people fret over points for style when they are going through tough times. I'd be lying if I said I didn't sometimes reach for a Snickers bar for consolation on a particularly bad day. But in the main, I stick to my healthier habits and healthier routines no matter what else is going on in my life. And the more you're in them during good times, the more likely you'll remain in them through bad.

A lot of this isn't just about routines and patterns—though a good portion of it is. Often you can "fake it 'til you make it." Stay true to your good routines even when your heart is not in them; eventually your heart will follow. But a lot of the problem starts with your mind-set. Between my mother's articulated preference for a daintier little girl and my own floundering, I quickly returned to a get-thin-at-all-costs mentality. And my eating habits followed. At least the rabbit part did. Then inevitably I felt hungry at a time of night when the only food available to me was junk.

The textbook definition of a compulsive eater is someone who binges but does not purge. Typically, these eating binges are driven by emotional needs. Compulsive overeaters eat because they're angry or lonely or frustrated. In addition to being genuinely hungry at night after eating so little during the day, I also ate for other reasons: I was angry about my mother's death, lonely even among peers at school, frustrated by everything out of my control, from my mother's death, to my body, to my eating.

Compulsive eating never satisfies a genuine hunger. Often the eating is accompanied by some other activity, like watching television. One minute you're vaguely thinking, "Oh, this chocolate tastes so good." Then you realize you've gone through five or six candy bars without realizing it. The food becomes its own distraction.

That was me again, back at school. I was eating without needing to. I was not eating when I was hungry. I can tell you if you don't know already, the self-loathing consequence of this kind of eating is scalding. It was particularly tough for me because I'd managed to break the cycle once, yet here I was again locked back in it. It had taken so much effort to change the first time, I couldn't believe I'd allowed myself to slip back. But that can tend to happen when we're under extraordinary stress and pressure. And that is why we need to redouble our efforts in better times and check ourselves with a special vigilance when times are bad.

6

Working It Out

Toward the end of my years at Kent, college came to be my ultimate goal. Gradually, I began to settle back into the healthier eating routine I'd initially established through crew. So I was feeling better again physically and I was even beginning to heal emotionally. It's amazing what time can do—even without any effort on our part. But like many of my classmates, I'd begun to hanker for a fresh start and a wider stomping ground. My problem was going to be how to pay for it.

Most of the kids at Kent came from wealthy families, so when my friends started looking at schools

the talk was usually about one elite private institution or another. My stepfather didn't have that kind
of money, but I talked the talk just like everyone else.
I figured—naively, perhaps—that I'd get accepted
first and deal with the tuition later.

I suppose there was something fatally unrealistic
about my approach, like I was setting myself up for
a fall, but I kept at it. I knew that the decisions I made
in the next few months would dictate the kind of
person I'd become. This was my future, about to
happen, and I wasn't about to screw it up.

For some months, I'd been thinking about a career in broadcasting. I was a complete "Tonight
Show" freak. I used to stay up late, drooling over
Johnny Carson's job. Really, I thought he had the
killer gig of a lifetime: to sit there, night after night,
making everyone laugh, meeting new people, learning about their lives. I just needed to figure a way to
get from my seat to his.

Syracuse University had a competitive rowing program, and one of the best communications schools
in the country, so I set my sights there. The only negative was that it was also one of the most expensive
schools in the country. Bill kept telling me to go to
one of the state schools back in Texas because it
would cost so much less, but there was no way I
could be in Texas.

My only chance of going to the college of my dreams would be through a rowing scholarship. It was the only way.

I soon became consumed by the idea of going to Syracuse. I just had to get that scholarship. It mattered so much to me. In some ways I think I'd simply transferred my desire for the perfect body to a desire for matriculating at the perfect college. In both cases, I genuinely believed that if only I attained my desired object, my life would be bliss. (Now I'm leery anytime I begin to get that if-only feeling again. It's a clear sign I'm veering toward an unlikely fantasy.)

But rightly or wrongly, Syracuse was the prize and my eyes were on it. I woke up each morning *praying* the mailman would arrive with news of my acceptance—and my scholarship.

One day, fortunately, he did. Thanks in large part to the efforts of my coach, Syracuse offered me a full-tuition athletic scholarship. So the following fall I headed north with great expectations.

Rowing at the big-time college level was a major adjustment from prep school. Oh, the sport was the same, but the competition was far more intense, and the effort we put into it increased exponentially. The coaches had us thinking crew was all that mattered. We rowed every morning for two hours, and every afternoon for another three. We lived and breathed and ate our routine.

The eating was a big part of it. We ate as a team, and we ingested thousands of calories every time we sat down, just to keep pace. It was eat or wilt. It sometimes felt as if we existed merely to burn energy and to refuel, which wouldn't have been such a terrible thing except that I was still prone to my own brand of emotional eating. And, I suspect, I still had enough of a negative body image to leave me insecure. The slightest thing—a depressing phone call from home, a bad grade—could set me off on a binge. But given the college crew schedule, I'd never notice the extra calories. I was working out like crazy, and my endorphins were sky-high, which helped to settle me emotionally, but also helped mask my feelings about compulsive eating.

I was on such a wild ride; by the time I returned to my natural endorphin levels, it was usually time to go work out again. I was all over the place.

I was still stepping on the scale regularly, but now the deal was to keep the weight on, not take it off. I wasn't supposed to dip below my prime weight— about one hundred sixty-five. It was a totally new mind-set, one I didn't adjust to all that well. I'd look over at my training partner, and see that she weighed a little less than I did, or maybe that she was a bit thinner in some areas, and I'd panic. What was she doing that I wasn't doing? What did I eat last night that I shouldn't have? Maybe I should work out more, or eat less.

One of the more curious side effects of my training schedule was the split personality I developed about my appearance. On a competitive level, I was almost arrogantly confident about the way I looked. I was proud of my body, and I loved showing it off to other athletes and coaches in a position to appreciate it. In my gear, out on the water, there was nothing I couldn't do. But on a personal, more intimate level, I was often embarrassed by the way I looked. For some reason, I still felt it was vital to fit into a pair of size ten Calvin Klein jeans. I just couldn't buck the culture. (This was just about the time a young Brooke Shields wouldn't let anything get between her and her Calvins.) My legs, abs, pecs . . . everything could be rock-solid perfect, but I'd still get crazy if my jeans were too tight.

My size continued to be an issue in my relationships with men. My freshman year was when that one guy told me that he was afraid that if I lay on top of him I'd squash him. It wasn't long after that I began dating only the bigger guys I tended to meet down at the gym. That's where I already spent most of my time and the kind of guys I met there tended to be more appreciative of my sport than others on campus.

Even then, I was often extremely uptight about my body. I find that somewhat ironic now; I don't think I've ever been in better shape or my muscles better honed. Sometimes my body made me feel sexy, even powerful. But usually, I felt more self-conscious than anything else.

For example, the very first time I was with a guy, I spent more time thinking about myself than I did about him. I worried whether my thighs were too big, or if maybe I should turn myself to the side a bit to make my stomach appear smaller. I was so caught up in lighting and body angles and how I might disappear gracefully under the covers that I never fully gave myself to the moment. Weird, huh? There I was, more naked than not, sharing my first intimacy with another person, and in my head it was all about how I presented myself to him. I was so caught up in not embarrassing myself that I forgot to enjoy what he had to offer.

Over time—thank God!—I became more relaxed in a sexual setting, but I was still uncomfortable on my own. I began to develop more confidence in my appeal for men—experience was a great teacher— but I continued to lack confidence in myself. And the root of my self-doubt still resided in my body. Even in top form, it remained the source of my low self-esteem. If I'd been given the chance to trade my body for a more mid-sized model, I would have! And I can say this even knowing how much I got out of crew, a sport I excelled at chiefly because of my size.

Low self-esteem can lead to other problems. My senior year, on St. Patrick's Day, I was out with a group of friends at a campus pub. We were drinking, having a good time. At one point, I realized I'd had a little too much to drink and decided to call it a night. I said my good-byes and headed for my apartment, on foot, alone. Halfway there, I started to feel a little woozy, so I stopped to rest on the back steps of a friend's building just a few blocks from where I lived. I figured if I nodded out my friend would be home before long and help me inside.

As it happened, another "friend" beat her to it, a guy I'd known since junior year. We were all part of the same social group. He'd been drinking with us at the pub, and had noticed me on his own way home, so I didn't think anything of it when he offered to help. That's just it—I didn't think. The next thing I knew I was waking up in this guy's bed, naked and horrified. I had no recollection of what had happened, but it was clear. I raced to the bathroom, did what I could to clean myself up, and got the hell out of there. I didn't even stop to tell this guy off.

I was mortified, embarrassed, and confused. Was it date rape? Maybe. Was it possible that I was too drunk to remember being a willing partner? Possibly. But either way, this guy took advantage of a bad situation. He was a shit, but I did nothing about it. I had such a low opinion of who I was and what I looked like, I was scared to make a fuss. Instead, I avoided the asshole for the rest of my time at school, thus keeping clear of any possible confrontation. I hated the way this incident would make me look if it ever got out, so I pushed it out of my head, for a time at least.

Plenty of other women who have been in similar spots have probably responded the way I did. Better to let it pass, keep it quiet. But the fact that I responded this way was significant to me because it was not my style. At least I didn't think it was my style. Yet there I was, taking it. Backing down. I didn't want to expose this guy for what he was because in so doing I would have had to reveal myself. And I didn't want anyone to take a harder look at me. I didn't want to take a harder look at myself.

I began to wonder if this would be my trend for life: back down, take it, don't stand up for yourself. It didn't feel like me, but I've always believed we're defined by our actions, not our opinions.

I was also beginning to burn out on crew. It was

taking so much of my time . . . but then it always had. The real issue was it wasn't working for me anymore. There had been a time when crew seemed to offer a solution: It gave me confidence, a source of genuine pride, and it also gave me more control over my figure than I'd ever had before. But it wasn't enough. I was still obsessing on gaining weight. I was still inherently dissatisfied with the body I'd been given—and I was feeling this way even though I'd shaped my body to its absolute best. I felt like I was looking for the wrong solutions. For so long, crew seemed to be making me a better person; suddenly I felt it was making me worse.

There were big ramifications for me if I dropped out of the sport. My scholarship would vanish. More importantly, I didn't think of myself as a quitter— much as I didn't think of myself as the type to remain silent in a case of near date rape—yet here I was again, choosing an option I didn't like to think was characteristic of me. But in this case, I truly felt I needed a clean break. More than anything, I wanted balance in my life. And crew is a sport of extremes.

I knew that if I stopped rowing, I'd be shutting down my high-calorie-burning engine. I would no longer be able to rely on rowing to maintain an ideal weight. I'd be an ordinary person again, fighting that familiar battle with my weight.

But I was also beginning to think of the future. It didn't take an astute observer to figure out that there weren't too many opportunities in professional women's rowing. I would have to find *something*. And soon.

I decided to return my senior year and put my heart and soul into it. The summer helped clear the intensity of the six accumulated years I had dedicated to the sport. I loved my team and saw that I had it in myself for one more year.

In essence, I began to feel my life needed some major overhaul. I had to break the cycle I was in. I thought leaving crew would help, but I'm so glad I stayed with it—it was my constant, my security blanket, so to speak. Change would come but not by quitting something that was so positive in my life. I had enough with my horrible relationship with food and how it seeped into various parts of my life. I believe this was a start for me to demand better of myself—I was at an all-time low and I think that is what triggered it to begin.

*P*ause

It's natural to want to blame someone else for our troubles, to hold others responsible—particularly if we've had a rough childhood. It seems fair and reasonable to assign blame: We wouldn't be so screwed up if only we'd been treated differently, if only so-and-so hadn't been in our young lives.

For a long time, I blamed Bill for my problems with eating and weight. I wouldn't have had such a negative attitude about my size without his influence. I wouldn't have suffered from such distorted eating patterns. Or so I used to believe.

Maybe Bill was to blame, maybe he wasn't. Maybe I would have wound up as I did even left to my own devices. Who knows! What's the point? I could spend the rest of my life wallowing in self-pity and self-righteous indignation, doing an archaeology of responsibility, ascribing blame. But what would that serve? Where would it get me? In fairness to Bill, I really do believe he meant well.

And he was certainly plagued by his own demons, his own obsession about his weight and his eating habits. A lot of the way he raised me had more to do with him than with me.

More to the point, if I believed he controlled my early years, why should I willingly give him the rest of my life? That's effectively what I would be doing by remaining a prisoner to his fears.

There's nothing to be gained by slipping into the role of victim as far as I can tell. It's one thing to try to understand how you came to be the way you are, to trace the roots of your beliefs, but only if you have a mind to change, to acknowledge the past but get on with your life. In other words: Look back but don't stare.

I thought I'd cast off Bill's influence by the time I reached college. Rowing gave me such a feeling of empowerment; even though my path was still a rocky one, I felt released. But in fact, I remained locked in his mind-set. And I was a prisoner by choice. I was using crew to achieve what essentially were Bill's ends—or at least the ends I'd long ascribed to Bill.

I hadn't lived under the same roof with Bill for years, but here I was all these years later, letting him live rent-free in my head. It was up to me to evict him once and for all. And as long as I con-

人

tinued to hold him responsible, I wasn't likely to release him. You can't let go and hold on. I could always keep blaming Bill, but I would still stand five foot eleven inches. I would still weigh one hundred sixty-five pounds. I could let myself be miserable, sustained only by the consolation that I knew who was at fault. Or I could simply accept that for whatever reasons, I'd reached this point. Was I going to stay that way or would I change?

I knew I wanted to change. I just didn't know how. I only knew what wasn't working. I'd have to chuck it and try something else. I was feeling so low I decided there was nowhere to go but up! That may sound very negative, but it actually was fairly liberating. I had nothing to lose. So I decided to think about my next move, then make it. I would concentrate on the effort, not the results. And if I didn't like where I wound up with that, I would try something else.

I know it's hard to be resilient. Believe me, when I was graduating from college, I wasn't this optimistic about getting to a better place emotionally every minute of every day. But when I didn't feel optimistic or upbeat in my gut, I still knew intellectually that taking positive steps in another direction was my only real option. And even when

I couldn't hang on to this concept intellectually, I still kept taking those steps.

Personal change and growth happen only when the pain of where you are is greater than the pain of change. I had definitely reached that point. In the words of some twelve-step groups, I was sick and tired of being sick and tired. I was ready to get well.

7

*P*erseverance

I was still very interested in a career in broadcasting. I was determined to take the initial steps that would ultimately land me a job in television. In my wildest dreams I still had my eye on Johnny Carson's spot, but I knew there were plenty of other realistic jobs that would be very satisfying to me.

I applied to WTVH-TV, Syracuse's CBS affiliate, for a summer internship following my junior year. It would be a start.

Sports was pretty much what I knew, so I asked to work in the sports department. Unfortunately, the sports anchor had this thing about not wanting a female assistant. Apparently there had never been a female sports intern at this station, and if I was anybody else I might have looked elsewhere, but I wasn't about to be turned away so easily. (Mom taught me the importance of equality.) I called the sports anchor directly and told him I'd like nothing better than to get him coffee all summer, and that I fully expected to be his first female hire. He laughed, but said there were no openings.

"Would it be all right if I called on you again?" I asked, not wanting to let this contact slip away.

"Be my guest," he said.

"Would the first of the month be too soon?" I wondered.

"Fine," he said, and from his tone I could tell he wasn't expecting to hear from me again, or ever to have to take my call.

As promised (threatened?), I called him the first of the month—for the next ten months, until he grudgingly offered me a job for the summer after my junior year. (Sometimes it pays to be a pain in the ass.) I made plans to work three or four days a week down at the station, while taking one course at school, and started to look forward to a pressure-free summer: no rowing, no worries . . .

The job started out pretty much as I had expected. There was a lot of coffee-fetching and Xeroxing in the beginning, but eventually I started doing some work in the editing room and covering some minor stories, picking up little snippets here and there. The grunt work never disappeared, but I made time to learn about reporting, editing and lighting sets. I asked the right people the right questions. And I got the bug. By the time school started up again I was convinced that a television newsroom was the place for me.

I started applying for all kinds of communications jobs, but in truth I wasn't qualified for any one of them. I couldn't afford graduate school, not that an advanced degree would have necessarily made me a better candidate. And I wasn't too keen on going back home to work some entry-level position in Houston.

A lot of my friends were in similar situations. We'd sit around late at night, bemoaning the unfriendly job market, trying to figure ways not to have to work for a living. A couple of us hit on the idea of heading out to California. It was a wonderful whim: If I wanted to pursue a career in television, there were worse places to be than Los Angeles. So after graduation, I made a beeline for the City of Angels along with a tight group of friends.

One of the first things I did in L.A. was chart a path to Johnny Carson: I applied for a job as an NBC page. I figured once I got my foot in the door,

I'd be guest-hosting in just a few months. In order to do this, though, I had to get past a woman whose job was to sit behind an enormous desk, smoking Carltons and intimidating the hell out of kids like me. She was in charge of the famous NBC page program, and she wasn't hiring. Yet.

In the meantime, I signed on at a neighborhood shoe store and bought into the lifestyle. I fit right in, right away. I treated myself to the best pair of roller skates I could afford and started zipping all over town. I didn't have money for a car or even a bike, and public transportation was a joke, so I needed some way to get around. The skates were a cool option, except when grocery shopping; then it got a little hairy.

God, I was happy those first few months out in L.A. It was sublime. I was living with good friends, having a blast and feeling pretty great about myself. I loved all the organic foods people ate out there, the way everyone was so attuned to their bodies. I loved skating to work each morning, selling nice shoes to nice people. I loved being in sunshine, being athletic in my own way, on my own schedule. One of the great things about L.A. was the way everyone out on the beach was just so incredibly healthy, and honest, and open to new ideas. People talked about their problems, without fear of reprisal or feelings of guilt or sadness. It was like a new dawn for me. There was a tremendous energy to the place, and my days were filled with hope and joy and possibility. Nothing could bring me down. All the mixed signals I'd been trying to process about the way I looked began to melt away. I wasn't thinking about gaining weight, or losing weight. I was eating what I wanted—what I felt I *needed*—and I worked out when my body told me to. So what if I was selling shoes for a living? I was living, that was the key.

Some months into my California idyll, I took a call at the shoe store from the woman at NBC. There was a job for me as a page, starting tomorrow. Was I still interested? I hung up the phone thinking, *Okay, my life is starting.* It was like the skies parted and the world was put on pause; I was about to enter the picture.

All that night, I felt that I was on the brink of something important. Some people think being an NBC page is the lowest of the low. In truth, it wasn't much better than being a tour guide at Disneyland or Universal Studios. We were paid next to nothing, and were treated like wannabes. But I felt it was precisely in the right spot, where I was meant to be. It was what I wanted—to be close to the creative process, to see television from the inside. I even loved the idea of having a uniform. Advancement could come in its own time.

As it turned out, I was right that my first day as an NBC page would be momentous. I was only wrong about the way in which it would be significant for me.

That morning, the page supervisors handed out uniforms in size sixes and eights to all the other girls. There was nothing for me to wear, not at first. Apparently, female NBC pages came only in sizes six, eight and ten—or, at least, most of them did, until I came along. Once again, I took in the message that I was too big, that I would never fit in. There was no room for me here.

My new friends recognized the indignity potential of the moment and told me I was better off not having to wear such a hideous outfit, but they still giggled proudly when they donned their uniforms. It was sweet of them to try to make me feel better, but the effort was transparent. The uniforms meant something to them, as surely as the lack of a uniform meant something to me. I wondered if there would ever be a place for me. It seemed like I was always almost *there*, but I'd never fully arrived. It wasn't just Bill. The whole world wasn't prepared to accept me as I was.

And then, something interesting happened. Something momentous. I got mad. Really mad. More angry than I've ever been. This was my I'm-mad-as-hell-and-I'm-not-taking-it-anymore moment. I didn't start screaming that from the rooftops. I'm sure my fellow pages and the page supervisors had no idea what I was thinking, and the anticlimactic truth is that someone eventually dug out a still-too-small size twelve for me to wear, but in the space between having something to wear and not having something to wear I was transformed. I was made aware. It was as if my whole life had led me to this moment and I finally got it: I wasn't wrong. I wasn't inappropriate. The world—from Bill to NBC!—was wrong for not accepting me. And I had internalized this logic. It was so much a part of me, I didn't need anyone around to tell me I was constitutionally wrong. Well, I wasn't going to be part of that status quo anymore! I was so angry with this sudden realization, I almost couldn't see. I felt dizzy, but underneath I felt empowered. And it wasn't just an empowering thing— it was emboldening. I knew I would live my life with a new strength from that point forward. The uniform, by the time I squeezed into it, was almost beside the point. The real point was that I had to make a place for myself; I couldn't sit around waiting for the rest of the world to let me in. I was like Dorothy in *The Wizard of Oz*, and there was nothing in the Wizard's little black bag for me. I would have to find what I needed within myself.

As soon as I got a chance I made my way to the "Tonight Show" set. It was early in the morning of my second day on the job. The set was empty. I stepped through the curtains to Johnny Carson's star, the spot downstage where he delivered his monologue each night to millions of people.

You'd have thought that the incident the day before would have left me feeling lucky just to be a page—that I should simply feel glad not to have been given the boot because I didn't fit the uniforms. But I still had that new vision. So I didn't just feel grateful to be permitted on the premises, I was still full of hope and determination, and still aspiring to Johnny's job. Maybe higher.

Pause

We are not second-class citizens. I can hardly believe this requires stating, but it does. Too much of the world is still stacked against us. We still are sent too many signals that we don't fit, we don't belong. It's up to us how we receive them.

We're more likely to change sooner than the

world does. So the onus is on us. The world is going to continue delivering that message: We're inappropriate. It's up to us to reject that message. We have to try not to let it get us down.

We probably can't work on the world—at least not quickly enough by my lights!—but we can always work on ourselves. It gets back to a question of attitude. Attitude can be cultivated. It can be shaped to suit our needs. Don't be afraid to talk to yourself. Sometimes you need a pep talk; who better to give it to yourself than you?

Don't hesitate to tell yourself that it's the other guy's thinking that is incorrect. Why are we so quick to assume we're the ones who are in the wrong?

Or look at it this way: Remember that sports anchor who made it a practice not to hire women? I'm sure you feel as outraged as I did whenever this sort of sexist discrimination goes on. Well, what if I told you he'd hired women, but only women who were size ten and less? Would you feel as outraged? You should. You should be mad as hell. And you shouldn't take it anymore.

In the real world, the message is far more subtle. Take those uniforms. The page supervisors were genuinely sorry not to have a uniform in my size. I could tell that they felt bad. But the message is still the same, even when it's cloaked in apology: *I'm sorry, but you just don't fit . . .* The intention may not be malignant, but the effect is still the same. So be on the lookout. Be vigilant. Until the rest of the world catches up to us, we'll have to continue to watch out for ourselves.

8

The Start of
Something Else

After about a year of giving backstage tours
and seating studio audiences at game shows,
I found myself thinking more and more
about getting into television news. Being an NBC
page was great fun, but it was mostly that—fun. It
wasn't exactly a job, and I certainly couldn't stay there
forever.

The way it works in television news is, you start
small and move up. For on-camera journalists, this
typically means a series of two-year hauls in pro-
gressively larger markets—moving from a city with,
for example, a choice of supermarkets, to a city with

an airport, to a city with one professional sports franchise, to a city with a choice of airports and professional sports franchises. After five or six stops you might find yourself in New York, Los Angeles or Chicago, if you keep advancing.

I sank all my money into a demo tape (a kind of calling card/audition), made forty copies and crossed my fingers they'd bring me some kind of return. I was scraping the bottom of my bank account, but I tried not to focus on that. To better my chances, I applied mainly to NBC affiliate stations, realizing that the network's Burbank address on the return envelope might leave more of an impression than my audition itself.

The strategy didn't exactly kill. Over the next few weeks, I collected thirty-eight rejections—and two offers! The news directors at NBC stations in Palm Springs, California, and Flagstaff, Arizona, found something to like enough in my tape to offer me positions as general assignment reporter. Palm Springs promised a life of sun and fluff, lots of celebrity stories and probably very little in the way of hard news reporting. Flagstaff was something else. It was unlike any place I'd ever lived. My maternal grandfather used to tell me we were part Cherokee, and now that I had the chance to live in that part of the country, and to learn about the Navajo and Hopi cultures, I jumped at it. If I was a bit more Machiavellian in my analysis, I would have seen that a job in a ritzy vacation destination, where Hollywood's movers and shakers occasionally looked up from their unwinding to watch the local news, would have been a better billboard for my efforts, but I didn't see it that way. Palm Springs would be a breeze; Flagstaff would be a challenge. I opted for the tougher ride.

I wanted to discover new things about myself, to push. It's possible I also wanted to get back to a state with a desert, to see if I could be happy there. So I packed my few belongings in a U-Haul, grabbed a cup of drive-through McDonald's coffee the next morning, and kissed California good-bye.

I swear, I didn't think I'd make it. It was the longest drive I'd ever taken, into the most unfamiliar environment I'd known. I was incredibly nervous, to be starting out in this strange new place, entirely on my own. When I finally pulled into town, I was horrified. All around me was this vast emptiness—the great outdoors! There was just one major strip, with lots of shopping malls and fast food places, and that was all.

I found an apartment with a local manicurist, who turned out to be one of my all-time best roommates. She taught me to eat potatoes and macaroni and cheese when times were tough. Unfortunately, times were tough right away. My salary was just shy of eleven thousand dollars, which even in Flagstaff didn't stretch all that far, even in 1987. There were some weeks when we didn't get much beyond starch with some steamed vegetables thrown in for color. I barely had money to gas my car—a beat-up Hondamatic "Green Pea," which I'd taken to fueling one gallon at a time.

Times were tough on the job as well. The folks at KNAZ-TV took a while warming to me. They saw me as a prima donna from L.A., with plenty of high-powered network friends. They were way off, of course, but that didn't prevent them from feeling that way. I was also about a head taller than everyone else. The on-air reporters at this particular station were all very short, with petite features, and I stood out like Daryl Hannah in *The Attack of the Fifty-Foot Woman*. My new colleagues accepted me in time, but I never lost that feeling of being outside the curve. Ironically, though, it was in television that I found my first level playing field: It didn't much matter if you were large or small, we all looked the same on the small screen.

It was a long time before I stepped back and appreciated that given my difficulty accepting my body image, television was an odd choice for me for a career. Given my frame of mind at the time, you wouldn't have thought I'd have opted for such a high-visibility field. To tell you the truth, I never made the connection. I'd like to think that somewhere deep inside me was a healthy self refusing to accept the obstacles to my career aspirations.

The one problem with my new job was that I wasn't very good at it. I had a hard time writing for broadcast. This was basic stuff, yet I struggled for hours with my copy. One time the news director actually pulled the pages from my typewriter and tore them in half. How's that for demoralizing the new kid? But she was right. The rhythm of the writing—and there *is* a rhythm to good broadcast journalism—kept eluding me. The news director tried to get me to calm down, to write the way I spoke, and eventually I caught on.

I stayed nearly two years—about as long as a reporter is meant to stay in a media market such as Flagstaff. In that time, I worked the general assignment beat, covering lighter, service-oriented features. I found I actually preferred the softer assignments to covering crime and local politics, although Flagstaff was such a sleepy place there wasn't much in the way of hard news. On the weekends, I hosted a talk show and had a chance to interview all kinds of interesting local people. I did the weather and anchored the local cut-ins during the "Today" broadcast. I did a little of everything, although I never got to anchor the news. For some reason, the people who sat in those chairs never missed a day.

The weather gig led to a classic mishap. I had to do my forecast in front of a giant magnetic map of the United States, and it took a few days before I was comfortable in front of it. In that time, disaster struck. I had to put little sun and cloud magnets all over the country along with the temperatures in advance of the newscast, then I'd refer to them during my segment. What I didn't appreciate was where I was supposed to stand in relation to the map. One night, I turned to gesture toward an incoming front and bumped into the map with such force that all of my little magnets fell down. It was quite a sight— and of course we were live. Everyone around me on the set was snickering, but I managed to keep myself together. I just looked at the camera and said, "Well, I guess the temperatures are dropping all over the country."

Other than being such a klutz, I was proud of myself for the way I handled my first big career debacle. As probably the largest weather girl they ever had, I could have dissolved into tears. That I made a joke of it instead was a sign to me of my increasingly positive attitude.

The "Today" assignment ran for several months,

and it was probably my highest-profile position at the station. I was living one of my dreams, but I was up with the roosters—at 4:30 A.M.! I may have looked great on camera, but with these hours my social life wasn't what it had been in California. It's somewhat unnerving to be a prominent person in a small town. Everybody seemed to know me, but I didn't know them. I never quite got used to it. I didn't think of myself as any kind of celebrity, but I suppose that's what I was. But it made me feel more distant from others than accepted.

You really have to love what you're doing to keep such ridiculous hours for such a ridiculously low salary and to move about in the bizarre light of small-town celebrity. I might have adjusted to the weirdness of being on television and perhaps even to my schedule, but the lack of money was draining me. I took a second job as a fitness instructor at a local gym just to keep up with the bills. I was working all the time, as much as seventy hours a week, and when I looked ahead to my future in television I couldn't see much beyond Flagstaff. Like everyone else in smaller-city television news, I had my tapes out and circulating in larger markets, but I wasn't getting any nibbles. Even if there were other prospects, I couldn't see another two-year hitch for next to no money in a slightly larger city.

What I needed was a plan. What I found was the germ of an idea. Since high school, friends had been telling me I should model. Strangers would sometimes tell me the same thing. I always took it as a great compliment whenever someone suggested modeling, but I never took it seriously. It seemed pretty far-fetched. I weighted about one hundred sixty-five pounds, and I figured I'd have to lose about forty of them—in the right places!—before any agency would even let me in the door. Anyway, I couldn't see the point. Who wanted to model? Back then I thought modeling was nothing. All you did was stand around and smile. Where was the challenge in that?

Nevertheless, while I was still in California, I let myself be talked into posing for some shots with the NBC staff photographers, thinking I would send them out and see what happened. I might have known what would happen. My head shots were great, but when the agencies saw the body that went along with it, they weren't interested. They were kind enough in their rejections: "You're not our type," or "You're not what we're looking for at the present time." I got the message: I was too big to fit their ideal. I was too tall, too heavy, too much . . .

I can't say I was surprised.

Before long, I heard about a new kind of modeling. A friend of a friend had just signed on with the prestigious Ford modeling agency in New York, in their large-size division. Who even knew there was such a thing? I collected the details like bulletins from the front: You mean I wouldn't have to lose any weight? They would take me as I am? And how much do they earn? I thought she was kidding. From an eleven-thousand-dollar salary, one hundred fifty dollars an hour looked like all the money in the world.

In the back of my mind I figured that since things weren't opening up on air I could try to segue into some kind of career in front of a camera. So that's just what I did—at least that's what I set out to do. I took a job as a secretary in a New York investment firm—at twice my Flagstaff salary!—thinking I'd use some of my downtime to look into this modeling deal and see if it might be for me.

*P*a u s e

I don't know why I never viewed my size as a reason to avoid a career on camera. I was determined to work in the field of my dreams, and I guess I just didn't look on my body size as any kind of deterrent. To tell the truth, I never even processed my goals in terms of how I looked. I simply wanted a career in television news, on air, and I was absolutely going to go for it, no matter what. For all my troubles as a kid, I was never a "can't-do" kind of person. I wasn't scared off by hard work or long odds. Such faith probably flowed from my early praise-filled years with my mother, and from crew, and from growing up in the desert. Whatever it was, I knew that if I stuck to it, I could make it happen.

I think it's important to understand that I didn't consciously defy common wisdom by seeking a job for which I may not have been outwardly qualified, but I do endorse the practice. If we're going to remove the yoke of society's concept of the ideal and the norm, we might as well start by rejecting its manners of measure.

You can start with your scales.

I used to live in terror of the scales. Between Bill's ghastly weigh-ins and the pressure of my weekly weigh-ins for crew, I had an unhappy history with measuring my worth in pounds. I can recall those times when tipping the scales by as little as one pound above a hoped-for weight could send me into a depression. The few times I hit my mark or weighed in lower, I was thrilled—until the next time I tipped the scales.

I know I'm not alone in this. I'm not the only woman whose spirits have been chained to her scales.

Why should we endow the scales with so much power? It's a measure, but only one measure—one that has taken on far too much significance in too many people's lives.

I no longer weigh myself unless I have to. And I no longer scrutinize my body in front of a mirror, obsessing over every "trouble" spot.

This doesn't mean I turn a blind eye to my body. I simply use a different measure.

My clothes and my energy levels are my best indicators of how I look to the rest of the world, and how I feel inside. I'm no longer vigilant about my weight, but I am vigilant about the two areas more directly in my control: diet and exercise.

If we truly are what we eat, then that's all the more reason to think hard about what we're eating. These days I eat when I'm hungry and my diet is rich in fruits, vegetables, pastas, rice, beans and breads. I've found that this is the fuel I need for my body to function at its best. This doesn't mean I never indulge in sweets and other high caloric treats, but I try to strike a balance. And I've also cut out caffeinated coffee, something I used to love.

In terms of exercise, I also try to strike a balance. I'm not obsessive about it and unlike in my crew days, I now aim for variety. Walking, biking, hiking, running, swimming . . . anything that gets my heart beating. I don't have to be a world-beater on the treadmill to see results, and I can miss a day (or three!) if my life gets too busy. The point is, I need to take my body out for a test run on a regular basis to keep it functioning at its best and to keep looking my best. Health and stamina are my goals, not an impossibly slim body.

I've learned to celebrate the simple strides I make each morning. If I can wake up early to sneak in a yoga practice, a walk or rollerblade before work; if I can walk past a coffee bar without a tinge of anxiety; if I can reach into my closet and know that last summer's bathing suit will still fit, then I know I'm doing okay. I also know what to do if I've gained some weight—without freaking out, thank you! If I'm on my program with respect to diet and exercise, I don't need to step on a scale, reach for a tape measure or give myself a degrading once-over in a full-length mirror.

Some time after I became a model, I made a promise to myself to reclaim my diet, to take the responsibility for what I ate back into my own hands. I threw out every diet product that had found its way into my home, and as I filled two garbage bags with "lo-cal" this and "fat-free" that, I felt a great weight being lifted from my shoulders. It was a very tangible thing, and yet at the same time I also felt afraid. I may have been on a destructive cycle with my eating habits, but it was the only cycle I knew. I dreaded the idea of going my own way, even though I knew I had to.

Well, let me tell you, this was the best commitment I ever made. I've since learned the pleasures of moderation. There are no such things as "bad" foods, but certain treats do need to be doled out sparingly and treated with respect. This thinking takes time, but I am finally free from the crazy diet mentality that ruled my eating habits from as far back as I can remember. It's enormously liberating, to be able to eat when you're hungry, and to be able to eat whatever it is that you're hungry for. When I was able to do that, I found I was fueling myself and not fooling myself with the foods I was eating.

And I *feel* a lot better about myself than I ever did when I knew exactly how much I weighed and exactly where that weight had concentrated itself.

Ah, the beastly bathroom scale, the source of

so much of my adolescent angst. When I was a kid, ours was state-of-the-art—one of those daunting medical scales you rarely see outside a doctor's office. It was worse than any imaginary monsters lurking underneath my bed. It was on this scale that I was subjected to constant weigh-ins by parents who charted my weight on a wall. I used to wish for an old-fashioned floor model, the kind with the uncertain, wavering needles—and room for interpretation.

It was strange how adolescence changed the way I approached my regular weigh-ins. The boys I knew had it easy. When they hit puberty, their weight gains were welcomed, even encouraged. But we girls knew how vital it was that we control our weight. Any measurable increase was a cause for alarm, especially as we matured. And it wasn't just our parents, selling us on this notion of maintaining an ideal weight; we sold it to ourselves. When we were weighed at school, we watched each other and compared. I know one woman who avoided the ordeal altogether; she was so much bigger than her friends that she couldn't bear to see it quantified, so she found reasons to stay home every time our physicals came around on the school calendar.

These days I see the same thing all over again

at health clubs and gyms. We should all know better by now, but we can't help ourselves. I keep an eye out, to see how people handle the problem that for so long handled me. Some won't wear so much as a towel when they step on, most likely out of fear it will weigh them down. Every woman has her little adjustment to tilt things in her favor. Some weigh themselves on tippy-toe, thinking perhaps this will make them lighter. Some stand all the way forward on the springy platform; others stand all the way back. I've seen some women exhale. And I can tell how invested they are in the scale's verdict. I see the way their faces brighten when the weight balances at an acceptable level or the way they step off with a look of such dejection you'd think they were just given six months to live.

I saw one woman weigh herself three times during one workout. Three times! She weighed herself on the way in, with all her clothing; she weighed herself naked, after her shower; then she weighed herself when she was dressed and ready to go. Each time, she approached the scale like it had something important to tell her.

I know that when I used to weigh myself at friends' houses, when I was still stuck in the drill, I worried constantly about the accuracy of the scale. I imagine most of us have done that, at one time or another. People keep their scales heavy, or light, and if you don't watch your step you can "lose" ten pounds on false pretenses. You'd "find" that weight soon enough. The whole experience was like being told I'd won the lottery only to learn the one-million-dollar prize would be split one million ways.

So here's my solution: Let's all go out and bury our bathroom scales and everything they represent. Why not? I'm talking about a full-blown funeral ceremony, with a eulogy and everything. Find a good spot, get out your shovels and really, truly bury these suckers. Get into it. Invite your friends, if they're caught in the same swirl. Come up with some appropriate final words, maybe even an epitaph for a headstone. The symbolism is important. After all, what do scales represent for most of us? Failure. And there's no better way to beat back failure than to put it where it can't touch us.

If you can't live without a scale, and I know hundreds of women who feel that way, buy a new one and let it represent a new approach. Use it as a tool, and bury the old scale with the old ideas attached to it.

I should have gotten rid of my scale long before I did. I certainly had my chances. With each move——to a new town, or a new apartment——I in-herited a new scale or I went out and bought my own. I don't know why I kept subjecting myself to the routine, but for a long time I really clung to this monitor. It was a long time before I found the confidence to trust myself, before I realized that all I needed was to put the right foods and fluids in my body, and keep an active lifestyle.

Today I honestly don't obsess about it anymore. Thanks to the resolve I have found in books and within myself, I've stopped the self-hating act of pinching my tummy and shaking my thighs to see if they jiggle or rub together. This is less a diet indicator than an excuse to drive yourself crazy. Instead of freaking out, I talk myself through whatever is bothering me. Don't kid yourself: Mind and body work very closely together, espe-cially in this area. Take the time to really think your troubles through. Write down your thoughts in a journal and refer back to them from time to time. I know that I sometimes took a lot of hos-tility out on my body, and it was only through thinking about it and writing about it that I was able to recognize it and work against it. Once you see your own patterns, you'll be amazed at what you can change.

I've now got my mind and body aligned to

where I can *feel* when I'm a little heavier than usual; I can *see* it in the way my clothes fit; I can *sense* when I'm not operating at my peak levels. I just know through learning to *trust* yourself, you will too. If you work with yourself, like I did with myself, you'll get to where you'll know what feels comfortable, what feels right, and you'll know what to do to turn things around. You'll know how to adjust your levels of stress and energy so that you can function efficiently.

Which brings me to one final point. If you do decide to chuck your scales and instead focus on proper diet and exercise, be sure to leaven your new regimen with a healthy dose of patience. Change is hard and real change—the kind that becomes habit—is slow. Patience goes against the grain of our instant-result expectations, but it's really what is in order here. And I know from bitter experience that if you don't bring patience to bear, you'll probably get frustrated and give up too soon. With the right amount of patience, you'll have time enough to accomplish anything.

9

Yes, I'm a Real Model

My move to New York City was very for-
tuitous in a special respect. The reloca-
tion afforded me the chance to reconnect
with one of my great college pals, thus beginning the
romance of my life.

Phil was a terrific guy. In college, we'd only ever
been friends—good friends, but there had never been
anything beyond friendship between us. After graduation we'd drifted apart. But I'd known he was in
New York and once I got there I looked him up right
away.

Phil was as creative, funny and dependable as I'd

remembered him. He was also cute, but he was about five foot eleven inches and maybe one hundred fifty-five pounds, tops. Clearly not a suitable frame for someone like me. Or so I thought.

This puts me in mind of another aspect of size discrimination. We can be as guilty of size discrimination as the rest of the world. I certainly was with Phil. Because he was only my height and so lean, I had taken him out of the pool of potential boyfriend material for me. Even when I began to feel attracted to him, I at first rejected the impulse. I just couldn't picture us together.

Phil actually had less of a problem with the size issue than I did. He was far more accepting of me exactly the way I was than I was of him! I'm happy to report, I got over it. Given Phil, it wasn't hard. The truth was, our bodies fit together beautifully— whether we were dancing, or walking down the street, or making love.

The more comfortable we became with each other, and with our friends, the more we challenged people's preconceptions of how couples "should" appear. There's no sport in letting those notions stand, and we didn't. We're about the same height, but I like to wear heels. Phil didn't care; he actually encouraged me. I even wore heels to our wedding, and he showed up with a top hat. I thought that was just perfect.

* * *

The more I looked into modeling, the more I realized I would have to start with one of the smaller agencies. In 1989, the plus-size industry was so new that most of the top agencies—Wilhelmina, Elite, Zoli—had yet to figure what to make of it. They were still sitting this one out. Even Ford didn't have much of a track record in it. But then I came across an article about one of the boutique plus-size agencies in town, one of the few outfits doing any kind of real business in the field besides Ford. According to the piece, the head of the agency was looking for new talent, so I pulled a Liz Claiborne pants suit from my closet, wrapped it with a thick patent-leather belt, slicked my hair back in a tight bun, and made plans to drop in during my lunch hour. I didn't tell anyone what I was up to, not even Phil; sometimes it takes the pressure off if you don't announce things.

I had no idea what to expect—no idea, even, what I was looking for. I suppose I just wanted to test the waters, see what kind of reception I'd get. I wanted to know if modeling was a real possibility for someone like me, before I invested too much emotional energy in the idea.

I stepped into a no-frills reception area, decorated with photographs of beautiful, large-size women.

The receptionist looked up to greet me. From the look on her face, it seemed not to matter that I didn't have an appointment.

"Oh my God," she said. "You're absolutely perfect. Don't move. I want someone to see you."

This was going well.

The receptionist sent out a booker—one of the industry's key, front-line professionals, who markets models to clients—and she echoed the receptionist's enthusiasm. This second woman explained that her boss was out to lunch, but should be back shortly. "Would you mind waiting?" she asked. "I'd love her to meet you. It'll just make her day."

Her day? What about mine? "Sure," I said, trying to keep cool. "No problem."

Come on, how often do you get to hear that you're absolutely perfect? I wasn't about to abandon this scene until I knew what it had in store. I waited only about fifteen minutes for the woman in charge to show up, but in that time I got a little carried away. I fantasized a superstar modeling career for myself. I sat there thinking, *Here I am, in a modeling agency, waiting to meet the boss.* This had started out as a cold call, and now I was feeling all kinds of heat. I think I was starting to sweat.

When she finally showed, the head of the agency was indeed intrigued by my appearance. I don't know that I made her day, but she definitely made mine. "Don't change a thing," she said, and in those four words I found tremendous validation. For the first time in my life, someone looked me square in the eyes and praised my body. This was no hollow compliment; New Yorkers like this woman don't have time for faint praise.

A part of me had always feared the day when I would see myself along the sliding scale of everyone else's expectations. And now this, at last. This woman looked at me and saw no flaws. I was exactly right. My heart soared. If a brief exchange with this woman could make me feel this great, then modeling would be a constant affirmation.

I had everything to learn about modeling, and no time in which to learn it. Worse, there was no one to teach me. The agency just threw me into it, which is the way it usually happens. The top photographers have a way of tapping into a model's sense of herself, of making her feel like she's the most majestic creature who ever sat before a camera, but I was at such a basic level of the business I didn't have much contact with that caliber of professional. As a result, I was pretty much on my own. I didn't know about posing or angles. I didn't know what to do with my hands. I didn't even know how to smile. I thought I did, but I was prone to these horsey, full-wattage smiles that made me look like Mr. Ed. In real life, it just looked like a basic smile, but in photographs it was too much. A professional model's smile is really more of a smirk, tinged with a grin and a knowing look. It's not a natural kind of smile at all, at least not for me. The big smiles were okay if we were on a beach, or romping through the autumn leaves, but to sell an elegant outfit you had to have an elegant, knowing smile. Mine needed work.

All I knew at the outset was how to pack my modeling bag—after I learned what a modeling bag was. The agency folks were kind enough to clue me in on this one. They told me what kind of makeup to bring (matte base, powder, eye shadow, concealer, lipstick, mascara), what kind of hose (opaque, sheer and knee-highs, each in tan, black and navy), what kind of shoes (black flats, black heels; brown flats, brown heels). They told me to pack dental floss, and cream for my legs, and a razor in case I had to do lingerie. And padding! This was the grand paradox of large-size modeling. All the girls wore hip-pads and butt-pads, from Frederick's of Hollywood, to make us look even bigger!

My very first booking was for a discount department store chain. They were shooting a circular for a Sunday newspaper insert. The client threw me in and out of five outfits in an hour. I had to wear these oversize polyester schmattes from hell, real house-dressy kind of stuff; if I'd stood anywhere near a cig-arette, I'd have gone up in flames. I earned one hundred twenty-five dollars for that first hour, and that's all it was—just one hour. It was like an assem-bly line, the way they had us running in and out of the dressing room, trying to get their money's worth.

I played it as cool as I could, but it was hard not to be wide-eyed. There seemed to be tremendous ex-citement and energy to the studio. I had about a mil-lion questions before we even got started, and a million more after that, but the answers had to come from experience. Until they did, it was downright embarrassing. On that first shoot, one of the girls suggested I practice moving and posing in front of a mirror for a while, to understand the angles of my face and body. I tried this and found it helpful, but nobody told me I had to *stop* moving for the pho-tographer to take the picture. Why should they have to tell me something so basic? I was a professional model, right?

Yeah, right.

It got to where the photographer's assistant actu-ally had to count out, "One, two, three, click," to cue me when the camera was going to go off. It was one step short of asking me to say "Cheese!" God, I was mortified.

With practice, my movements in front of the camera have definitely improved, but back then I thought I was hopeless. It's a wonder I ever got a second assignment.

From the moment that booker told me not to change anything, it was as if the world tilted on its axis and there was room for me. Even though I'd been heading in the right direction in terms of self-acceptance, I have to admit this was a clincher. I'd been talking a good game but now when I passed a mirror I honestly felt great. For some reason, my acceptance as a plus-size model struck me as the ultimate validation. Fortunately for me, my thinking didn't stay this way too long.

One thing about the modeling business: Even though your looks are your livelihood, you have to develop a pretty thick skin about them pretty quickly. On assignments, I hear unflattering comments about my appearance tossed around all the time. It's nothing personal. Sometimes I'm just not right for a certain job. (Luckily, I'm right enough most of the time—right enough to make a living!) For me, hearing myself discussed so frankly so frequently has been the ultimate liberation. I never put too much into any one comment. From experience, I've learned that today's verdict is sure to be overturned tomorrow.

So, perhaps ironically, modeling has led me to the truth I've suspected all along: My sense of self-worth has to come from within. It can't be anchored to an aspect of myself as variable as my weight. It's been a long path with what may seem like a self-evident truth, but it's one thing to appreciate a truth and acknowledge it, it's quite another to live it and feel it in your gut.

Through modeling, I've also learned another truth I could have suspected: Plus-size women aren't the only ones who are prisoners of poor body image. Plenty of "straight" models—models size six to eight—are as insecure about their bodies as I'd long been.

Sometimes I wonder about all the collective energy, effort and worry women direct toward their figures. Just think what we could achieve if all that effort was directed elsewhere. We are physical beings so we will always need to take care of our bodies, but there's a difference between healthy maintenance and obsession, between balance and extremes. If I had one hope for us all it would be that we find that balance, that appropriateness. And then we could direct all that leftover energy and effort to endeavors that will really make a difference—in our lives and in society.

* * *

Early in my modeling career I developed a strong feeling that the Ford agency was where I wanted to be, much the way I'd once set my sights on Syracuse and later NBC. I had to work up enough of a portfolio to impress the folks at Ford. After about six months of steady work that included my first national ad, Ford finally took notice.

It was through Ford that I collected my first location assignment. It was for a major southwest department store chain called Foley's; the shoot was in Texas. The client flew us down to Houston, and then we drove out to Laredo.

Everything's always six months ahead in modeling; in summer you shoot winter, in winter you shoot summer, to accommodate the long lead times of most catalogues and monthly magazines. So for this particular assignment, we were shooting a winter catalogue in the heat of summer. We stood in the middle of a buffalo pasture, sweating like crazy in our woolen knee-highs, thick corduroys and cowboy boots, trying to shake a colony of red ants from our clothing. It was about one hundred and ten degrees, and there was no air conditioning in the van, and no water to flush the toilets. It was so hot we couldn't keep our makeup on.

I'll never lose that image of me standing in that pasture, dressed for winter while the heat rose from the dry plains, trying to maintain some dignity posing next to a herd of buffalo. So much for the glamorous world of big-time modeling! But I earned good money for my efforts (two full days of pay, plus a half-day of travel).

That first location shoot was also memorable because it placed me back in my stepfather's orbit. I had put off telling Bill about my modeling, and when I finally got around to it he seemed unmoved. He hardly ever told me he was proud of me, or that he thought I was beautiful, or that it was a good thing large-size women were being depicted in such a positive way. Nothing. And yet when I stopped in for a surprise visit on my way back from Laredo, I was treated to a heartening surprise. There, on Bill's coffee table, was a pile of my magazines, laid out for any visitors to see. I could have cried. I'd always thought the reason Bill never said a word to me about modeling was because he didn't care, and yet he cared enough to collect my magazines and leave them on display. Family friends had always told me Bill was proud of me, but I'd never seen any evidence of that. Here was the confirmation I'd sought from him for so long. If only he'd been able to tell me more directly. But that just wasn't in the cards. From talking to friends, I know that many parents seem to have a tough time expressing approval and giving praise. Yet those same parents may be the biggest braggarts when their kids are out of earshot. What a shame for both the parents and their children that the joy of such accomplishments can't be shared.

Pause

Seeing those magazines on Bill's coffee table was a nice moment for me, but my greatest sense of satisfaction from modeling came from the fact that a body like mine can be out there as an alternative to the ingrained ideal that has had such a lock in the media for so many years.

I still often get incredulous looks when I tell people I'm a model. They look me up and down and think I must be kidding. You? A model? Well, yes. And a *real* model, to boot, representing more than sixty percent of American women. Large-size modeling is still in its infancy, but we are slowly gaining visual acceptance in the advertising community—and I hope by the public. I wonder if things might have been different for me if I had been able to se a body like mine in advertising and the media when I was growing up.

I ask this question because it distresses most of the young people I talk to about body image and fitness almost as much as it distresses me. I'd say about ninety percent of the fifth to eighth graders I've met are concerned about the ways they are being represented in the magazines they read and the television shows they watch. "No one looks like me, Emme," I'll hear. "Why don't we see larger girls in *Cosmo* or on 'Melrose Place'?" "How can I feel good about myself when everyone is so much thinner?"

It's tough, I know, but we have to work through the prevailing ideal and hit upon one of our own. Or, we can come to accept that we will never see our true reflection in the mirror of the mainstream media. It would be easy to point the finger at Hollywood or Madison Avenue executives, and to criticize them for presenting such an unattainable model, but the burden is really on us—on parents and kids alike—to sift through the impossible images and accept them for what *they* are, not for what *we* are not. Let it be up to us to reject the impossible in favor of the possible. Let us decide our own taste, and our own fate.

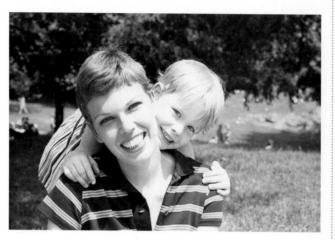

New York's Central Park, 1968: Me, age 5, with my mom, Sally. Mugging for the camera came pretty naturally to me.

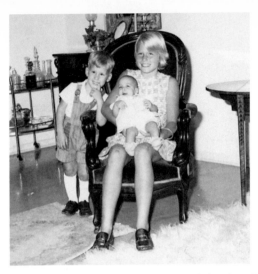

In Dhahran, Saudi Arabia, 1972: Me, with brother Chip and baby sister, Melanie.

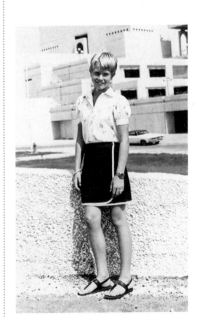

1974: At age 11, I was a tall, athletic kid who was put on the scales more than often enough.

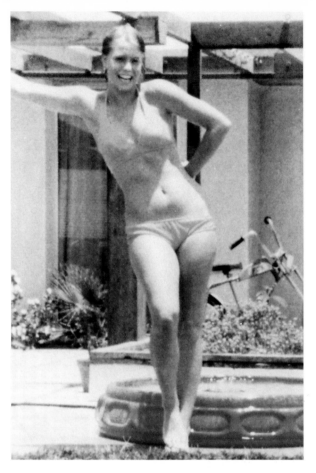

Around the pool in 1976: Thighs too big. Waist too wide. Stomach not flat enough. The image I had of myself at thirteen was pretty distorted. Today, I can love this body and I appreciate the great, young healthy body it was.

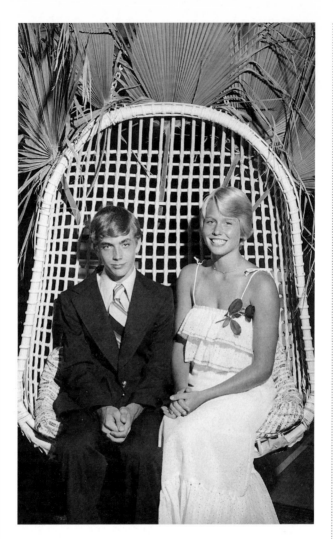

Unlike so many of my peers, I was taller than my date. And, judging by this photo, considerably more mature and poised.

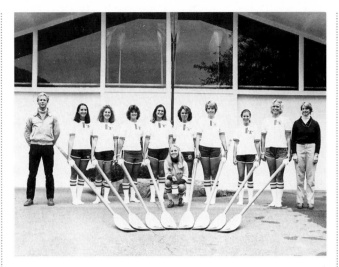

The Kent School Crew, 1979 (me, top row, second from the right): For the first time in my life, my size was an advantage. That big smile was hiding a lot of pain, however, as I wrestled with a lot more than a few extra pounds.

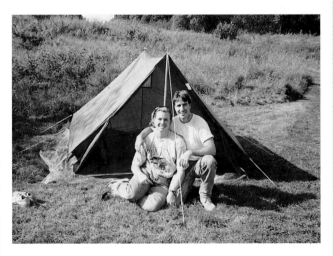

My life isn't all glamorous locations and photo shoots. Here, with my husband, Phil, camping at the Allagash Waterway in Maine, 1991.

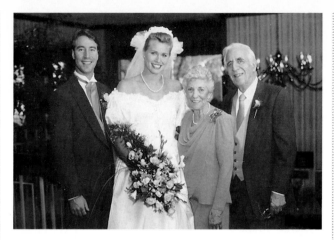

Our wedding, November 12, 1989, with Phil's grandparents.

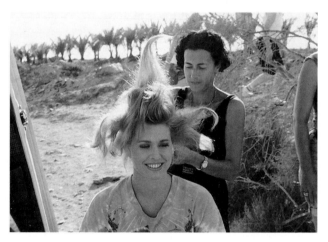

Getting teased! On location in the Canary Islands, 1992.

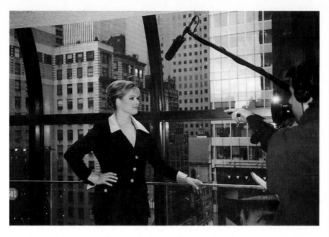

At the celebration for my Times Square billboard, New York City, 1996, being interviewed by E! Entertainment TV.

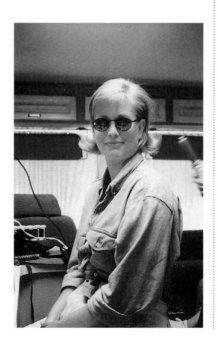

Miami, 1995: Waiting—and waiting and waiting —in the motor home before a shoot.

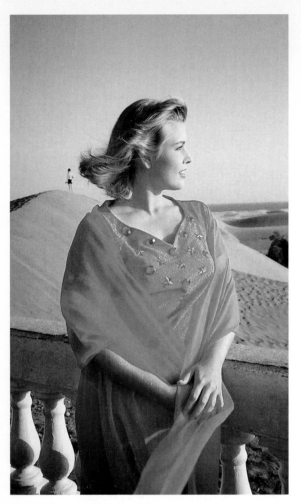

On location in Las Palmas, 1992.

The fashion industry excuses itself by explaining that fashion is fashion, and that it is merely good business sense for them to display their wares on the most attractive bodies they can find. That's no excuse, but from an insular perspective it is all the justification account executives need. Yes, they'll argue, we want to sell dresses in size ten or twelve or fourteen, but if our product looks best on size four or six then that's what we're going to put in our ads. You paint a house before you sell it, right?

I can understand their point, but what *we* have to understand is that fashion is not reality. They're selling a fantasy, to go along with the clothes, and once we accept this as a given we can begin to accept the hard sell for what it is, and begin to feel a bit better about ourselves in the bargain. There's an obligation, I think, to look out for our young adults, and to keep them from feeling manipulated by the image makers, but if advertisers and media honchos won't assume that responsibility, then we'll just have to do it for them.

It is my hope that the proliferation of large-size modeling, and the wide acceptance of highly visible alternatives to the prevailing notions of feminine beauty, will help us to see a range of "preferred" body types in our magazines and on television. To my mind, such a flowering will signal true liberation from the tyranny of the slender ideal.

Several years ago, a non-model friend of mine was asked to participate in an article titled "The Great American Body" for *American Health* magazine. My friend was one of five female athletes (recreational, not professional) selected. The other women represented a range of sports—and a range of body types. There was a very tall, broad-shouldered cyclist, a short racquetball player, an aikido devotee of medium build, a swimmer, and an ectomorphic runner whose body most closely approximated our culture's ideal.

The point of the article was that there is no singular "Great American Body." The women featured were all healthy and vibrant but only one had a body that conformed to the type you're likely to see in most advertising. Each woman in the article was an appropriate weight for her frame and body type.

I believe this is the direction in which we need to head: toward a zeitgeist that embraces a multiplicity of body types rather than insisting on a singular ideal—an ideal that will remain inherently unapproachable, let alone unattainable, for most.

If you want to aim for an improved body, if you want to work toward an ideal through sensible diet and exercise, I urge you to fix the appropriate "ideal" in your mind before embarking on your plan. (I even hesitate to use the world "ideal" because I resist its implied singularity.) Figure out which is your Great American Body. Accept the reality dictated by your height, your frame and your body type. Try to value the type you are. Appreciate the strengths and, yes, the beauty. If we fail to identify that appropriate "great body" before "going for it," we will be doomed to failure and the gnawing recriminations that tend to result.

10

Showing My Stuff

In January 1994, the editors of *People* magazine decided it was time to feature a plus-size model in their annual survey of "The 50 Most Beautiful People in the World." What a fantastic notion—and clearly long overdue. That a magazine as popular and mainstream as *People* was looking our way was strong indication of a changing climate. I was thrilled.

Word got out quickly that *People* was looking for a plus-size model for the issue. Selection in this annual issue had proved to be a career-maker for a handful of previously unknown "straight" models, so the news created quite a buzz throughout the plus-size industry.

The magazine's editors started asking to see our portfolios. They asked questions: Would we be available for promotion? Would we talk about our lives for publication? Would we consider posing nude?

My bookers at Ford were ecstatic when I made the first cut, but I held back. *People* magazine? Me? One of the fifty most beautiful people in the world? Before I let my emotions run away with me, I reminded myself that I was still quite a long shot. I was also a little anxious about this nudity business, but I figured that *People* magazine was unlikely to veer from policy and feature full-frontal nudity in its pages. Besides, I'd done lingerie shots before, and that wasn't very difficult.

Still, I was barely prepared when I got the good news: *People* had chosen me!

I showed up for the shoot in a robe and thong underwear—hoping that I wouldn't have to reveal absolutely everything, but trusting the process. Theo Westenberger, one of the top photographers in the business, wanted me to pose as a reclining odalisque. She sent me upstairs to make up, and after a while she walked in and looked me over. "Emme," she said, "you're gonna have to take everything off."

"Okay," I said, cool as I could, "no problem."

Then it hit me: *They're talkin' nude, Emme. We're nude here; totally nude; nakednakednaked.* It was one thing to put on an intrepid front, but quite another to step out of your last piece of clothing in front of a roomful of strangers—however flimsy that last piece of clothing might have been. I wondered if I would have minded less if I'd been a more classic beauty, but I was far *more* than a classic beauty.

Anyway, I slipped out of my thong, took a deep breath and walked onto the set naked as the day I was born. It really wasn't such an ordeal, once I got into it; actually I put it out of my head. The set was closed to all but essential personnel, and everyone was so wonderfully supportive and over-the-top enthusiastic about the way I looked that I couldn't help but get into it. And it was all very dignified. I had my hair pulled back in a braided, beaded and oiled configuration, and I was stretched out on a divan covered with silk sheets and luxurious pillows. I felt totally sensual, and absolutely at peace with my body. I was transported to another time and place. I completely forgot that there were a half-dozen people milling about, worrying about the lighting and the set. There were even space heaters nearby, to keep me warm, and I forgot about those as well.

Three hours later, I stepped into the quiet of a February snowfall and could feel the flutter of butterflies in my stomach. I remember thinking the snow was sent to ease my transition back into this modern world.

I had no photo approval, just a few Polaroids to confirm that everything had been handled in a tasteful and elegant way. I took them home to show Phil. He was pleased with them, but I don't think either of us fully realized the impact it would have when the magazine hit the newsstands. We tried not to think about it. A couple of months later, on a Thursday afternoon, the editors sent ten advance copies to our house and we tore into the package like it was Christmas. We opened the issue on top of the pile and there I was—reclining provocatively across a two-page, full-color spread, an ostrich-feather duster dangling at my side.

I almost didn't recognize myself.

And get this: It wasn't enough to riffle through one magazine. We had to rip open every last one of them, and each time I saw my picture I was floored. Oh, my picture had been in national magazines before—I'd even been on a few covers—but this was something else. This was me, abundantly nude, in a magazine read by almost everyone I knew. This was me, in doctors' offices and airports and supermarket checkout aisles all across the country. This was ME!!!

I have to say, it was a sensational shot—a full-back

nude with a side glance over my shoulder—and I was deliriously happy with it, but this was the first time it really registered what I'd done. (Oh my God, what *had* I done?) I was naked to the world, completely out there, showing my stuff. Theo Westenberger had really done an amazing job in capturing the true beauty of the feminine form, but I couldn't shake thinking that I had just shared an intimacy with millions of people.

Phil and I flipped through the pages of those advance copies so many times we could have cooled the entire neighborhood with the breeze. Then we ran out to all the newsstands in town, to buy them off the racks as they came in; some we grabbed by the bundle, as they came off the trucks. It was absurd. We wanted to have enough to send to all our friends—as if they couldn't buy them themselves.

It was a heady moment. The neatest thing was to look at my page among the celebrities. My spread was right after Vice President Al Gore (Al Gore!), just before NBC News personality Matt Lauer. Joining us were Meg Ryan, Antonio Banderas, Denzel Washington . . . Yikes! I looked at all these beautiful people and marveled that someone had thought to include me among them. The accompanying article was also a surprise—I'd bared all, in an emotional sense. I'd talked frankly with the reporter and knew that everything I said was for the record, yet I was still surprised by what the magazine picked up on. The brief piece on me mentioned the frequent forced weigh-ins I'd endured as a kid as well as my lifelong struggle with accepting my body image. It was jarring to see myself doubly exposed, but I felt good about being in the pages and good about going on record.

I threw myself a party to celebrate the event. Friends and family came to my house in New Jersey and we sipped champagne and laughed at the serendipity of it all. Phil even had a blow-up poster made of my two-page spread, and he put it up in our hallway for everyone to sign. It was a perfect freeze-frame to a nice moment. Somehow, I knew my life wouldn't be the same after this issue had come and gone, and I wanted to hold onto that threshold while I could.

The magazine forwarded hundreds of positive letters from its readers, most of whom were grateful that someone of my size would share her story and express herself so freely. Two of these letters even made it into print in a subsequent issue. One, from a reader in Terre Haute, Indiana, put me back in my place: "Art collectors may appreciate a naked

Emme, but the average American wants to see faces, not fannies, in this issue. I guess I should be thankful it was her and not Al Gore."

Oh, well.

I was completely unprepared for the avalanche of attention that followed. There were requests for interviews from dozens of television and radio programs and national magazines; clients were suddenly hot to work with that plus-size girl in *People* magazine; women's groups wanted to know about my lecture schedule. Everybody claimed to have a new angle on my story, but the cumulative effect was consistent with the simple, positive message that had accented the "50 Most Beautiful People" spread: Feel good about yourself, no matter your frame. With each story came proof that people needed to hear what I had to say.

The letters continued to pile up—from all over the world; from young adults to great-grandparents; from housewives to high-level professionals—and it became clear in the rereading that I was onto something. There were women out there in a great deal of pain, desperate for a practical, positive body image to which they might aspire. I heard from men too, who recognized in me a kindred spirit and an emblem of hope. I even heard from people on the job—

makeup artists, other models, stylists, especially those who were maybe a little overweight, working in an industry that perpetuated an unattainable ideal while dealing with body image issues of their own. Many of my behind-the-scenes colleagues thanked me for shining a light on our shared concerns; many more told me they kept a copy of the magazine at home, for inspiration.

I decided to make a proactive effort to shake up some of our ideals, to challenge some of our widely held notions of what was beautiful and healthy and good. I put together a presentation on body image and self-esteem for high-school students, and made the time to visit some of the schools in my area. I pitched myself to talk show producers and seminar organizers and when I was invited to talk, I made sure I used my time to full effect.

I was in this frame of mind, going through this process, when my path crossed that young woman's at the intersection and I decided to write this book.

It was time for me to articulate the message. At least I could try.

Pause

Are our concepts of beauty changing? Possibly. Ten years ago, *People* editors probably wouldn't have run a spread of a large naked woman, albeit a model. Ten years from now . . . who knows? The real triumph will come when such photos appear without raising too many eyebrows—or if they do, it will only be because the model is naked, not because she is large.

True acceptance of other body types will be achieved when they appear in ads and don't stand out so much because they are such exceptions. I wonder if I will ever be able to appear in an ad next to a "straight" model without gaining any more notice than, say, a blonde model next to a brunette.

I don't mean to make too much of advertising, but ads do remain an accurate barometer of society as a whole. Acceptance in the media can both signal change and usher it in.

I am proud to say I happened to be a part of an unremarkable opportunity this past spring of 1996. I appeared side by side with my straight-sized counterparts on huge billboards in Times Square. The Liz Claiborne company devoted a whole block of billboards to their campaign: I was modeling for the company's Elisabeth label. I loved the attention it drew. It caused quite a stir, because it was the first time a large-size model ever graced Times Square. To say the least, I was honored to be a part of it. However, I look forward to seeing this happen as a regular occurrence instead of a rarity for plus-size models in campaigns to come. There are quite a lot of women who relate to us, the numbers are there, not to mention the spending dollars. Speaking of hoopla, what about the press coverage about a black and a white model sharing the cover of *Sports Illustrated* magazine that same winter? What was all the fuss about? Why shouldn't a black and a white woman stand together on one of the hottest covers of the year? No one probably was complaining about the onslaught of press coverage the girls and the magazine received. Let me tell you, as we change our views, advertising will have to as well. Change is coming, and it's about time.

11

Confidence

Have you ever known someone—male or female—who exuded a special radiance, a confidence that seemed to emanate from the core of their being? They had "it"—a bounce to their step, a genuine upbeat attitude. On closer inspection, that person may not have been any more attractive or any brighter than the next guy, but because of that innate sparkle, they radiated a special appeal.

Conversely, you may know someone who, although quite attractive, seems to give off a negative energy. That negative charge may come from a negative opinion of oneself. And while that opinion may not at all be based in reality, the effect becomes real enough.

While the person with that special air of confidence may seem to have had it since birth, that may not be the case at all. That kind of confidence comes from attitude. And attitude is like physical fitness: It may take time and effort, but it is definitely something you can acquire. Don't think for a minute that those who exude confidence don't still have to work at it. We do! Like the athlete in training, we need to work on our attitude on a daily basis. We're as human as everyone else.

And speaking of attitude—I've got a friend, Suzanne, who's been blessed with a great one. Actually, it took her a while to develop it, and she developed it out of necessity, but it keeps her sane and healthy and happy.

Suzanne was an athlete in high school, and a nutrition major in college, so she was more attuned to her body than most people are. Before she got out of school, a knee injury changed her diet and exercise habit such that she went on a new regimen and lost a great deal of weight. She found that she enjoyed the way people responded to her new physique. Her body wasn't crazy about the idea, but Suzanne liked her new look, and after she launched a successful career as a model, she was determined to keep it at all costs.

Well, let me tell you, it nearly cost her everything. She was so thin that even her modeling agency wanted her to gain weight, but Suzanne wouldn't listen. She was five feet ten inches, about one hundred and ten pounds, and she was inordinately proud of the fact that she could fit into size-four pants. "To succeed as a model, you had to stay thin," Suzanne explained to me when we sat down to talk about the hard turns of her life and career. "At the time, I would only eat fruit during the day. Just fruit. I knew I should be eating, I had the right instincts, but I also wanted the recognition. I denied myself because I wanted to succeed in this business. Modeling was all I had."

As it happened, Suzanne developed a blood disorder, and the resulting treatment transformed her appearance—and threatened her career. "I had to cancel all the work I had lined up in Europe," she recalled, "and check into the hospital. They put me on a steroid, and in just a few weeks everything changed. My body, my face, everything. I had this moon-shaped face. I couldn't even look in the mirror, it was so painful, and when I was finally well enough to go back to the agencies and see about returning to work, it was even worse. These people hadn't seen me looking like this. I was the same me, just bigger. I felt deformed. I was embarrassed. I felt like I had to explain before I even got there what the problem was, why I looked the way I did, but even after my explanation I'd still get these looks. People were just so unaccepting. I'd gone from a perfect size four or six to a bloated size ten or twelve. There was no way they could send me out on a modeling job."

Suzanne eventually returned to the industry as a large-size model, and she has harnessed her obsession with weight and exercise to where she is now in control. "My mantra now is, if you don't like the way I am, that's your problem, not mine," she revealed. "I'm not gonna change any more for anyone. My health comes first in my life right now. There's more to my life now than worrying about my dress size, about what I'm eating or not eating. My life is about how I treat other people. It's about self-love. It's about being a good friend, a good daughter, a good mate. If you're happy with yourself, it's gonna come through in your smile. It's gonna come through in your eyes. You're gonna radiate that."

Now, that's a positive attitude! But how can you work to develop your own? First, try to get a sense of where you are on the attitude continuum. Are you already fairly upbeat and confident? Or does the negative view come to you more naturally? Like most people, your attitude probably varies from day to day. But where would you say you are with the most consistency?

If you tend to be more negative, if you feel there really is a dark cloud over your head, that negativity may spring from low self-esteem. It can become a self-protective impulse. Because you don't think well of yourself, you don't think you're deserving of good things. So rather than set yourself up for disappointment, you set your expectations low. Expect the worst, then you'll never be disappointed. What you may not realize is that those who expect good things help make those good things happen just by virtue of expecting them.

I'm not talking about winning the lottery here, I'm talking about instances where other people are involved. Positive people tend to be very appealing. Think back to that person you know who radiates confidence. How do you feel when they enter a room? When they call? Their positive energy influences those around them. It informs the way the people around them behave toward them. So you literally can influence those around you just by radiating that same kind of confidence.

So how do you get that confidence? I can suggest a few steps that may bring you closer than you are now. Give yourself some time, but be sure to try to use these tools on a daily basis.

Talk to yourself. Don't be afraid to give yourself pep talks. I talk to myself all the time: before I go on a modeling assignment, when I have to speak to the media, when I have to meet someone for the first time. Talk out loud or talk to yourself mentally—although if you talk out loud you may want to make sure no one's in earshot! What should you say? It depends on the circumstances. If I'm being considered for a modeling assignment, I tell myself, "You're right for the job. They'd be lucky to get you." If you have trouble praising yourself, do a little role-playing. Be your own personal coach.

I also talk to myself afterward. If I didn't get that modeling assignment, I tell myself, "It's okay. You weren't the right match for that one. It doesn't mean you're wrong for everything, just this one."

Don't be shy about talking to yourself. Even people at the top of their game do it. During the 1996 summer Olympics, one of our top gymnasts was known for talking to herself before each performance. You could see her on camera, lips moving, reminding herself of critical moves and what she had to focus on. If gold medalists can do it, we shouldn't be slow to follow their lead.

Remind yourself that it is a level playing field. Sometimes in talking to other plus-size women, I get the feeling that many of us feel we have a unique lock on low self-esteem, acceptance of our body images and anxiety when it comes to everything from shopping to dating. While these issues may be problematic for us, they are also problematic for most people, no matter their size. It's not as if the rest of the world is operating at one hundred percent all the time and we're the only ones on the planet who are deficient. This point may seem so basic, but haven't you sometimes felt that you were totally alone in having to contend with such deficiencies? You don't need to be a plus-size person to lack confidence or have moments of keen self-doubt.

I have a friend who is a runner. One winter day she was running a race. It was already snowing hard by the time the race got started; there were several inches of slush on the ground and the footing was slippery. My friend was actually in the lead with about a mile to go when she began to panic: The course was just too slippery, she'd never be able to stay ahead, other runners were sure to catch up. Then she reminded herself that everyone in the race had the same footing to contend with. It wasn't as if she was the only one running in snow. She laughed at herself at how silly she was being; she couldn't believe she required a realization to appreciate so obvious a point. But I bet many of us have made comparable false assumptions. I know I have. Haven't you ever felt like you were the only one negotiating tough terrain, that for everyone else it was smooth sailing? Yet like that runner friend of mine on that day, we're often all on the same course. We're all human, all prone to the same insecurities and doubts. If we're large, or we have trouble with our weight, that's just the route those doubts and insecurities will use to get to us. If it weren't those areas specifically, there'd be other ones.

So tell yourself, no matter what doubts you're entertaining, you are definitely not alone. If you could read minds, if you could know the doubts those around you were nursing, your reaction would probably be, "That's so silly! How can you possibly feel that way?"

So why do your own insecurities somehow hold more validity? The answer is, of course, because they're yours. And since they are yours, it's harder to have perspective on them. So try to take that step back. Pretend you're someone else reading your mind. How do you view your insecurities now?

Think about your posture. Your posture can definitely influence the way you feel. If you don't believe me, stand up. Pick your chest up, pull your shoulders back. Don't think Marines, just relax and stand up straight. Take a deep breath. Exhale. Now take another one. Don't you feel better already? What were you so worried about just a moment ago?

Good posture can be particularly tough. My mother always told me to stand up straight when I was young. "If you're going to be tall," she used to say, "be proud of it." It wasn't easy, but I tried to follow her advice, and today, from a healthier, adult perspective, I understand her point exactly. When I see friends who slouch and try to "camouflage" their body, I can't help but think how terrible it looks. You might as well take out a billboard telling everybody how embarrassed you are by your appearance. And worse, when you slump like that, you feel terrible too. You may not even appreciate where it's coming from, but believe me, when you slump like that it puts your whole soul in a slump too. No matter how tall you are, you will look and feel better with better posture.

Try to catch yourself at different moments during the day. Whenever you think "posture," take a mental snapshot of how you're sitting or standing at precisely that moment. If you're like most people, it's probably not a pretty picture. So right after you take that shot, try to straighten up. In the beginning, don't be afraid to look in a mirror. When most people start to improve their posture, they worry that they are starting to look like some kind of recruit for the military. But by checking yourself out, I think you'll discover that what may initially feel like ramrod posture really is just putting you at your best.

Breathing. I mentioned breathing earlier, but it's worth highlighting on its own. Breathing brings oxygen into our systems. It is how we get energy, by oxygenating our blood.

If you're feeling down or anxious, give yourself a moment to take a deep breath. Inhale through your nose and keep breathing in until you feel your chest and even your belly expand. Now exhale slowly through your mouth. If you're still feeling anxious, breathe this way again. It has a great calming effect and will also serve to put you in mind of your breathing at other times. (Yoga is the best teacher for breathing.)

Déjà vu all over again. If you're like most people, the same kinds of instances probably consistently make you nervous: a job interview, a blind date. Every time you go through it again, you're probably as anxious as you were the last time. This is very natural. It's to be expected. But try to draw strength from the other times you've successfully sailed through such situations. Remind yourself that you've done this before. Remind yourself of the previous particulars. You may still feel nervous, but with luck and practice, you won't feel that overwhelming, defeating kind of anxiety.

I'm sure you'll be able to come up with other tools to use toward developing that positive attitude. Just remember, attitude is not like climbing a mountain. It's not like you reach a certain plateau and then you're there, always at that level. Think of attitude like fitness. You need to get your attitude in shape, then keep it in shape. Be prepared for setbacks, but continue to work consistently. Make the effort, then leave the results to themselves!

*P*ause

When I travel—modeling, lecturing, *listening*—I hear a lot of anger from many of the women I meet. There's also pain, and grief, and denial. It's a recurring theme: We seem to want to blame someone for the way we are, to absolve ourselves of all responsibility in our personal dramas, to hide from our problems with such elaborate deceits that we no longer recognize where we came from or where we're going.

This is not a good thing, but it is all around. I should know. I heard this anger in myself, for a time: I denied who I was, grieved for the person I would never be and blamed everyone and everything I could think of for my loss. It was a demoralizing way to live, so I worked to find a more balanced view. I'm still working on it, but I've finally gotten to where I can (and must!) take responsibility for who I am, and how I am, and why.

It would have been easy for me to blame my parents for instilling in me all these conflicted emotions about food, to look at my growing up as a kind of blueprint for a lifetime battle with my weight. Or, I might have pointed to genetic disposition, and cursed my parents for even thinking to bring such a big-boned child into this world. (How *dare* they consign me to such a fate?)

I used to keep a laundry list of reasons to explain away my circumstance, but the liberating truth was that there was never anyone to blame, not even myself. It took a while to realize that I could talk myself into feeling guilty, or I could rail against Bill's weekly weigh-ins, but that in the end all of this finger-pointing would have accomplished nothing. I would still stand five feet eleven inches, I would still weigh one hundred ninety pounds, and I would still be unable to find a decent outfit to wear to a party.

Were there things I would have done differently? Moments I longed to rewind and erase from memory? You bet—and then some. Yes, there were some messed-up notions around my family dinner table; and yes, if my stepfather had offered some consistently positive feedback about my appearance in adolescence I might never have developed some of the compulsive eating habits or negative body imagery that kicked in once I left home; there's even a good chance that if I had been born to more diminutive parents I'd possess a more diminutive set of genes. Who knows? Any number of things could have fallen a different way, but if they had, I wouldn't be the same person inside. This is my body, and this is my family, and this is my story. It all goes hand in hand with who I am today, and I can't change any one element without changing the whole. That I won't do.

I like who I am. I like that I can find something to laugh about in the darkest situation. I like that I can help make people feel good about themselves. I like that I've been able to surround myself with dear, loving friends. I like that I can confront my fears and meet my goals and move about with confidence. I like that my body is fit and toned, that I can stand in front of the mirror and find something to celebrate. (Finally.) I've learned to like the way I look—I truly have. I may not like a lot of the ambivalent stuff that went on when I was younger, or some of the ways my body responds to certain moods and hormonal changes, but these are things I've been able to get beyond. I can say today I am thankful to my parents for doing the best job they could at the time. Lessons were learned—big time.

I wasn't so accepting of my circumstances as a young girl, but I came to it in time. You can too. Accept responsibility for who you are, and who you might be. You can only blame your parents (or your metabolism, or your environment) for so long before the holes in your thinking turn up bigger than the logic behind them. Stop buying into your excuses and start believing in yourself. Invest now to get beyond what is holding you back— your future is waiting!

12

On the Road (Again!)

Like many working women, I travel a lot. In fact, I spend so much time on location shots that I'm constantly fearful of slipping into bad habits—or letting the carefully cultivated good ones fall away.

There's no getting around it: Routines, like Broadway shows, are tough enough without taking them out on the road. And it's not just the unfamiliar surroundings and schedules that throw me. I find there are more temptations outside the house as well, and more opportunities *not* to take care of myself. When I'm in a strange city, waking up in a strange bed, ad-

justing my body clock to a strange time zone and re-
lying on the sometimes strange foods found in airports and hotels, everything tends to just go out the
window as far as my diet and exercise are concerned.
Nothing is easy, and even our best intentions have a
way of disappearing. I know mine will if I'm not
careful. It's especially difficult to eat right, to find
time to work out or just to relax and let go of the
troubles of the day.

This unfamiliarity affects women of all sizes (and
men, too!), but it doesn't have to be a bad thing. Indeed, I've worked to make it a blessing. I've had to.
Most people are able to write off their occasional
travel lapses as blips in an otherwise healthy routine,
but I'm in too deep for that. You see, I spend about
one hundred nights each year in hotel rooms around
the world, and I simply can't afford to let myself go
for such huge chunks of time. No way. I'd be out of
a job and out of my mind so fast I wouldn't know
what hit me. I couldn't shelve my good habits every
time I left home without having to play some serious catch-up every time I returned.

Thankfully, I've come up with a few tricks to help
me cope, to make myself at home away from home,
and to create the kind of environment I need to stay
at my best, and I want to set them down here so you
can adapt my ideas to suit your needs. In some ways,

I've tried to use my time away from home to work even harder to give my body what it needs. And why not? When I'm done with my work, there's usually no one around to help me fill the rest of the day. There are no errands to run, no chores to do, no friends and family to visit, so I might as well put the free time to productive use.

I'll admit it now, I am obsessed with water and what it does *for* you. I will go into more detail later, but I'd like to share how it extends to my traveling fitness program. I am an absolute water hound. I spritz it on and drink it down and just relish having it near. I also swim in it every chance I get—*particularly* when I'm away from home. No matter where I'm going, I pack a suit, goggles and cap. I go on the assumption that I'll be able to use them, and I almost always do. Most of the better business-oriented hotels have indoor swimming pools on the premises, and when there's a pool around I know I'm in good shape. I usually look for accommodations with an Olympic-sized pool so I can do my laps, but any pool will do. Even if you don't swim strongly enough to enjoy the full benefits of a lap workout, you can put together a wonderful half-hour routine of leg-lifts, kicking and resistance training that will leave you feeling toned and refreshed. I know many women who never take advantage of their neighborhood pools, but who swear by their hotel sessions. After all, how often do you get to roll out of bed and right into your own swimming pool? (Okay, so I'm not counting the elevator ride down to the locker room, but you get the idea.) Take advantage of the proximity, and the time on your hands.

And speaking of time, a half hour is really all you need. At least it's enough time for me; if you need more time, find it. I try to wake up an hour or so before my first appointment, to leave myself enough time to get in a swim and to eat a relaxed breakfast. I don't like to rush things in the morning. If I've got a six o'clock call, or earlier, I'll save my workout for later in the day; I can't show up for a shoot looking exhausted, because that would kind of defeat the point. It doesn't matter if you're a fashion model or an account executive or a local sales representative: A good night's sleep—every night!—is a key component to any healthy travel regimen. Fresh air is another. The stale, recirculated air of most convention centers and hotel conference rooms can leave you looking pasty and worn for weeks after you return home. Get outside for at least a few hours each day, even if you're up in the mountains in the middle of winter. (Hey, especially if you're up in the mountains in the middle of winter!)

Swimming isn't the only exercise option, it just

happens to be my favorite. In addition to my swim gear, I always pack a pair of comfortable cross-training shoes, a headband, a leotard, a jog bra, a baseball cap, and a sweatshirt for cooler climates. I'm ready for anything. I'll sometimes go for a good brisk walk or hike around the area, or rent a mountain bike and tour the local hillside. If I'm in a downtown center, or out by the airport, or in a place that doesn't feel too safe, I'll look for a treadmill, or a stationary bike, or an indoor track. I've even found that in some of the bigger hotels in some of the bigger cities I visit there are hotel-sponsored running or walking groups that leave the lobby together each morning. This is not just a safety issue for me, it's motivational. It's so much easier to work out with someone else, even if it's a complete stranger—and there's no better way to meet new people than to run side by side with them through a new city. Ask at the front desk.

Safety can be a real concern, so if you're walking or running alone it's a good idea to let someone at the hotel know where you'll be going, and for how long. I've gotten into the habit of leaving my key at the desk, and asking the person on duty to recommend a good route, so someone will know exactly where I am. Lately, I've been running with a set of dog tags around my neck, preprinted with my name, home address, emergency contacts and medical information, in the unlikely event that I should drop into a ditch on the side of some running trail in the middle of nowhere. You can have your own tags made through ads in the back pages of most outdoor fitness magazines. In fact, you should. If you're like me, you probably never think of such precautions when you're exercising at home where you're known, but when you're out of town and on your own, they're doubly important.

Some hotels offer morning stretch or aerobics classes, or a staff trainer to walk you through any unfamiliar equipment in the gym. (Once again, seek and ye shall find!) Others offer shuttle transportation to affiliated local health clubs, where classes might be offered at reduced rates (or no charge at all) to hotel guests. It's usually a good idea at check-in to find out what services and facilities are available in and around your hotel and to plan your exercise strategy accordingly.

When I'm planning to be away from home for an extended period of a week or more, I'll turn my hotel room into my own personal gym by packing along one of those hard rubber flex-a-balls you see advertised on late-night television. They're a great help in maximizing sit-ups and push-ups and all kinds of calisthenics. They pack flat, to about the size of a paperback book, but when you blow them up they're about as big as a beach ball. It's a bit of an effort (and a lot of hot air!) to blow them up, but the results are well worth it.

If at all possible, I'll ask for a room on a top floor and take the stairs when I'm coming and going, just to get my heart pumping the way it should a few times a day. I'll even leave time in my schedule to walk to my appointments, instead of taking a taxi, if that's what I feel my body needs. The whole point is that it takes an extra effort on the road simply to match the efforts made at home, and I find I have to be creative and vigilant about staying on my game.

Of course, none of these extra efforts would amount to much if they weren't complemented by a healthy diet, and this too takes some work. A lot of times, when you're on the run, the only restaurants available to you are of the fast-food variety, but most of the national chains offer a salad bar option, or at least a few low-fat items. Check them out. And stay away from the fountain sodas if you can; I usually ask for a glass of seltzer, which is almost never on the posted menu but is almost always available. (The fountain sodas are a mix of flavored syrup and carbonated water, and most soda machines have a special button for seltzer; plain old water is also an option, although some places have the nerve to charge you for the paper cup.)

You can pretty much count on finding a piece of fresh fruit, a nice hunk of fresh-baked bread or a fairly good plate of pasta to hold you over until you can find a decent meal. The idea is to avoid the bad stuff while you're out scavenging for the good, and this is sometimes easier said than done. If you're at a morning conference, for example, or a large-scale meeting—or, in my case, at a catered photo session—you'll probably encounter an elaborate tray of danish and fruit; in the afternoon, you might find some cheeses and crudités. Lean toward the fruit and vegetables, and be leery of the sticky sweets and high-cholesterol items. I don't know about you, but if I'm not careful, I can just pop those cheese balls and doughnut holes into my mouth all day long, so I find I'm better off avoiding them altogether. Know your limits, and your tendencies, and keep them in mind.

These days, most hotels offer a mini-bar fridge stuffed with overpriced liquor and snacks, and these present a great opportunity to eat healthy foods right in your own room. No, I don't drink or snack to anything resembling excess, but I do empty out the mini-bars and use the refrigerator space to store things like celery, carrots, apples, yogurt, juices and my ever-present bottled water. (If you do this, make sure to return the hotel's merchandise to the fridge at the end of your stay or you'll be charged for it!)

With all this attention paid to smart eating and exercising, I sometimes feel I deserve a treat, so I try to pamper myself on the road. If there's a masseuse associated with the hotel, I'll be the first to make an appointment. There's nothing like a vigorous massage to get my mind and body on the same page, or to help me unwind at the end of a long day. If there's a sauna, I'm the first one in. I prefer a nice steam sauna, where the air is moist enough to open my passages and to do wonderful things to my complexion.

And my pampering extends to delicious treats—especially if there are local delicacies to be savored. Understand, I don't overindulge myself, but I feel free to sample, because I'm keeping my body in the same kind of balance that I do at home. A little ice cream or chocolate is not enough to upset a healthy balance.

For too many women, leaving home for a few days can be an excuse to break the good habits they've worked so hard to develop, but as far as I'm concerned it's no excuse at all. Slipping back into a positive routine after succumbing to the negative impulses of a prolonged business trip can be extraordinarily difficult, so why put yourself in that position?

Remember, every good habit we break is twice as hard to develop a second time. Stay the course, even when there's a change in scenery.

Pause

There's a lot of sitting around and waiting in the modeling business, which is great if you want to catch up on your reading but lousy if you want to stay in shape—and we *have* to stay in shape to stay in the business. What I'll try to do when I'm on a trip with a few other models is arrange some sort of evening activity like a group swim, an aerobics class or a long walk from the studio back to the hotel.

Things don't always work out as planned, however, and at these times we have to be especially resourceful. Once, on a shoot in Bremen, Germany, I was holed up in a wonderful old hotel with four or five American models for an entire day with absolutely nothing to do but watch German television and eat German chocolates. Let me tell you, it wasn't long before I had enough of each (oh, the chocolates were sensational, but there can be too much of a good thing). There was a torrential rain outside and our shoot had been canceled, and the hotel, despite its charm, offered nothing in the way of exercise facilities. We had to do something, so a group of us put on our workout clothes and hit the stairwells. To be sure, some stayed behind to finish off the chocolates, but that was their business.

It was a five-story hotel, which presented a significant challenge at a good pace, and we ran up and down those stairs for about half an hour. Some of the hotel guests and employees were looking at us kind of funny, but we didn't let it get in the way of what turned out to be a pretty serious, major-league workout. We were all sweating big time by the time we were through, but more important was the way we felt inside for having made the effort.

The benefits of hard stair work have been well-documented—just count the number of Stair-Masters at your favorite gym—but the added benefit here was the proactive interest we took in our health and well-being, and in each other. We felt sensational when we were through, and we had a complete blast.

What I learned on that rainy Bremen afternoon was that nothing worth doing comes easy. It's one thing to go to the health club, or to buy the latest piece of workout equipment for the home, but it's something else entirely when you have to make do with what you have. I learned that I must take my exercise where I can find it, because it doesn't always find me.

13

Fit or Fat?

Every now and then when someone I just met learns that I'm a plus-size model, they'll say, "But you're not fat!"—as if I'm somehow fraudulently passing myself off as a plus-size model. I explain that I *am* a plus-size model, that plus sizes are anything size twelve and above. I am not a model or poster child for obesity. While I advocate acceptance for body types, shapes and sizes that vary from the ideal or "norm," I am not a proponent for obesity. So I'm not pro-fat. But if I'm not pro-fat, it's more from a health perspective than a cosmetic one.

Whatever I do, I know I'm going to be big. That's

a given. Nothing I do is going to make me shrink below my five-foot-eleven-inch frame. Only a truly extraordinary and probably unhealthy effort is going to shift me much below my normal weight. But when I'm overweight, I don't feel my best. I don't look my best, either, but I hate the way it makes me feel more than I hate the way it makes me look. I feel tired. Draggy. I feel depressed because I know I don't look my best, because I have looked better. If I'm overweight, I am probably not keeping up with those exercise activities I have come to thrive on, activities that tend to elevate my mood in a healthy way (a balanced amount of endorphins): walking, hiking, biking.

You'll need to decide what's right for you with respect to fat, what is acceptable and what isn't. Whatever you decide, I urge you to accept your body type. And I encourage you to work toward health.

A friend of mine likes to say that he's a spiritual being going through a human experience. I like to think of life that way. It puts an emphasis on my spirit and soul while at the same time not denying the all-too-human aspects of being human. That includes being human in a physical sense. Like it or not, we're stuck with these bodies—at least this time around. I believe we need to take care of them. We need to make the most of them in that we shouldn't allow them to drag us down. We shouldn't be prevented from pursuing our dreams, our happiness, because we feel too tired. If our bodies are too fat, they're going to be working against us. It's up to us to take them back.

I really believe that a lot of the lack of success many of us have had with dieting comes from holding on to that inappropriate ideal. Even if we make some headway on a diet, chances are we're still pretty far off from the "straight" model ideal. So let me make a few suggestions:

1. Stop dieting! Now. Commercial diets have approximately a ninety-eight percent failure rate, so why undertake a program that will more than likely leave you no better off than when you began? After all, you wouldn't bet on a horse with odds like that, so don't start betting against yourself.

2. Learn to accept yourself as you are. If you have to aim for an ideal, make it one that is appropriate to your body type, your height, and your frame.

3. Aim for health and fitness in your eating habits and exercise plan rather than an "ideal" weight or an "ideal" shape. Think about getting your body to serve you in your everyday activities. Think about longevity. If you're feeling tired and

draggy now because of your weight, how are you likely to feel five years from now? Ten years from now? Twenty?

From personal experience, I know that it's a lot easier to start to feel better physically and mentally after only a week or two of exercise and proper diet than it is to feel like you're really slimming down. So stay attuned to how you're feeling, not how you look. If you stay on your program, your looks are likely to follow. But don't obsess about them. Take it a day at a time. A walk at a time. A visit to the health club at a time.

Personally, I don't believe in diets. Period. I've found the best way to lose weight is the slow way: sensible diet and sensible exercise. By definition a diet is something you go on and probably can't wait to go off. If instead you concentrate on sensible diet and sensible exercise, you're likely to come up with a livable lifetime program. The changes in your weight and your muscle tone may come more slowly than some of the promised returns of any diet, but chances are the results you do earn this way will be more sustainable—particularly if you try to craft a healthy program for yourself as a way of life, not just some temporary, probably desperate, solution.

Pause

Not every full-figured woman is going to have a career as a plus-size model, just as most "straight size" women will never grace the cover of *Cosmo.* So why can't non-modeling large women feel as acceptable as their non-modeling straight sisters? The sad fact is that straight-size women don't feel acceptable either. When you think about it, as I have, you'll see that on the most fundamental levels, we're all in the same soup together. Low self-esteem, eating disorders and low body images grow across all sizes in our society.

Modeling, for me, has been a tremendous boon. There's no denying that. Yes, I could have made a living doing any number of things, but this is what I chose to do. (Or, perhaps, this is what chose me.) But modeling is not the point. The point is that modeling facilitated my personal growth in an accelerated way. The point is that you are the only one who can change the course of your life, even as you stop and ask for directions. The point is that it's up to you to kick-start your own growth spurt.

I might have found this same perspective without modeling, but it would have taken time. You can find it too—in your own way, on your own clock. We can all learn from each other. I learned as much about true beauty from the straight-size girls in the dressing room as the large-size girls, but even more from the non-modeling crew. That's always the way of it. Throughout my life, the most dramatic lessons have almost always surfaced among my friends. We take from each other and give to each other to where our collective experience can stand as the model.

I've always felt that the lesson has never been so much in the lecture as in the example. I'm a *show me!* kind of person. You can tell me any old thing you want, but I'm not gonna buy it until I can see it for myself, maybe even try it on for a bit. A lot of people are the same way. I learn best from those who strive for the best, and I try to live my life knowing others might be traveling in my wake.

I tell parents all the time to listen to their kids, and to set the right example. Teachers too. I remind them to watch what they say, to say what they mean and to put what they preach into practice. How destructive is it to hassle your child about her weight when you yourself weigh more than you should? What student will really hear what you have to say about not smoking if he sees you lighting up in the teachers' lounge? How much credibility can you hope to carry with your adult children, in a discussion on the importance of the institution of marriage, when you've already been divorced three times? What kind of damage do we do when we don't learn from our mistakes? And where would we be as a society if we didn't seize on our neighbors as a resource and offer ourselves in return?

I think back to that adolescent girl I introduced in the opening pages of this book, the one at the local junior high school with the six-pack of diet-supplement drinks at her hip. She was there to teach me. I wholeheartedly believe that this girl was there to put me in my place, to challenge me to confront some of the issues that were keeping me up at night, to shake me from complacency into action. She was there to get me thinking about ways in which I might build on my position as a large-size model and my experiences as a large-size teenager to reach out to young people struggling with weight-related issues.

We find inspiration in the unlikeliest places, as

well as in some of the likeliest ones. The trick is in knowing what to do with it—and how to repackage it and send it back out there so that it might inspire someone else. That, I believe, makes the world go around!

14

What to Wear

We are all built differently. My measurements are forty-one inches by thirty-three inches by forty-four inches, and I fall somewhere between a standard size fourteen and sixteen. I carry my weight fairly evenly over my frame, in a fairly well-proportioned way, so what looks good on me won't necessarily look good on all of you, or vice versa.

But we can still learn from each other. Here, then, are a few basic things I think about when I put myself together each day . . .

Makeup

I like to wear my makeup as unobtrusively as possible, to make a statement without saying too much. This is a personal choice; you may choose differently. But in my view, it's always better to err on the side of too little makeup rather than too much. Your makeup should highlight your features, but it shouldn't be the first thing people notice.

If you need hands-on help with your application, you don't have far to look. Think about having a makeup party, where you and your friends can take turns applying and receiving different makeovers. Or take a trip to the mall. Most major department stores offer free or inexpensive makeup consultations to their customers, and you should take advantage of them to sample different foundations and colors, and hear what the resident "experts" have to offer.

The foundation is key. I think of it as a canvas, onto which I can apply colors to my various moods. Learn which of the four basic skin-tone categories (yellow-orange, red-orange, red and red-blue) you fall into. It took me a while to find a foundation that works consistently for me, to even out my skin tone. Now that I've found it, I rarely stray from my two basic shades—one for when I'm tanned and one for when I'm lighter. (Good news for African American,

Latino or Asian American women: Makeup lines like Iman's offer eighteen bases for darker skin!) Tip: Always apply sparingly with a sponge—not hands—the oils on your fingers can alter the color of the base foundation.

You can sometimes pick up free foundation samples, and don't be afraid to be greedy: The only way you'll learn to apply your makeup properly is through trial and error, so you might as well experiment. Keep in mind, though, that department store beauty consultants are also salespeople, so trust your own instincts; better, go with a good friend and accept what she has to say. If you feel pressured to buy something, make sure it's something *you* want, and not simply something the store is promoting.

I tend to prefer earth tones for eye shadow: taupe, beige, vanilla, butterscotch yellow, saddle brown, sometimes a mossy green. I like a natural, earth-toned four-color palette. I used to buy blush in shades of pink, until I picked up a few tricks from the pros who work on me each week. Now I've discovered that taupe is an awesome makeup tool. It can contour the face and lend great definition. It's also great around the eyes (in the creases, especially), and along the jawline.

Here's a tip: Underneath your cheekbone, apply a stroke of taupe from the very top of the bone near your ear, to the apple of your cheek. Then apply a lighter color on top of the bone (camel, perhaps) to accentuate your cheekbones.

Remember to blend as you go along. The most natural look can have a lot of makeup behind it, if it's done well. Treat yourself to a good set of brushes (blush, powder, lip, eye and eyebrow), and experiment.

A lot of women have trouble with their eyebrows; they shade them in or draw them two shades darker than necessary. Try to match them to your hair color; use a pencil for a natural line, then find a corresponding shadow to use as a filler. It's less harsh than using a pencil alone.

I wear a variety of colors on my lips. If I'm going out to a dinner or party, I might put on some dark red lipstick with a glimmer gloss over the bottom lip, or a pearl lipstick lined with a lip pencil, but even there I tend to prefer a clean, natural look of just a hint of color as a highlight.

Probably the most organic, energizing element in my makeup routine is water—as a liquid to drink, as something to splash on my face and as ice for a facial pack. (I told you I had a love affair with good old H_2O!) When I'm on the road with an early call, I'll run to the hotel ice machine first thing in the morning and treat my face to an ice pack for fifteen minutes or so. My earliest calls clock in around four-thirty A.M., and I'm not good for much of anything at that hour. The home-away-from-home–made ice packs ease the bags under my eyes and reduce early-morning swellings. I also drink tons of the stuff, wherever I am. I drink about ten eight-ounce glasses of water each day—even more when I'm traveling. Those airplane cabins can really dry you out. I wind up running to the bathroom all the time, but my body needs the extra fluids; my skin shrivels up without it.

Water even has a place in my makeup bag. I carry a little spritzing bottle, and use it to give myself a makeshift facial whenever I feel the need. Mineral water is great, but simple tap water will do. I also carry lipstick, Chap Stick, mascara, a tiny eyebrow pencil and a hint of cover-up for those breakout days, but the water is the one staple I can't do without.

Day or night, and from one day to the next, I try to mix things up a bit with my color combinations. You'd be amazed at the number of people who make themselves up the same way every day. Why is that? We don't wear the same clothes every day; you don't always do your hair the same way; there's no good reason to go out with the same face. If you've got sensational eyebrows, call attention to them from time to time, but vary your approach. Some people have wonderfully translucent skin, and they wouldn't want to slather too much panstick or makeup base over such a pristine canvas, but there are some occasions when a little makeup can go a long way. Try something new. Match your eye shadow to the color of your blouse or dress. The element of surprise can be a compelling accessory—and it can put some fun into your morning routine.

Perhaps my very best accessory is my confidence. Perhaps it's yours as well. We've already established that true beauty comes from inside, and it can radiate through the way you apply your makeup (if you choose to wear any), the way you carry yourself and the way you wear your clothes. It's all about presentation, and if the complete package reflects how you see yourself and how you want the world to look back at you, then you're ready to meet any challenge.

Clothes

You'd think a model would love to shop for clothes but I have to confess it is not one of my favorite activities. Truth is, I hate it! Particularly when I'm looking for something formal. I actually ache at the thought of finding just the right dress, at a price I can afford. I know women of all sizes have the same anxieties, but it seems an unusually troubling challenge for us full-figured women. In the past five years many department and specialty stores have expanded their lines to include plus-size fashions. There are probably more choices now than there have ever been, yet I still leave the house thinking I'll come home empty-handed.

Before setting out on a shopping expedition, you might take a look at what you have. If you're like me, your bedroom closet says a lot about how you once wanted to look, and very little about where you are today. Mine has "yard sale" written all over it—at least it did before I treated myself to a long-overdue wardrobe makeover. Believe me, it was an impulse born of embarrassment. A women's magazine sent a crew over to photograph my closet for an upcoming feature, and I was mortified at what they found. Those good people actually cleaned cobwebs from some of the back shelves, and rearranged all of my shelves and hangers. As soon as they left, I took a hard look at what was in there. I took out absolutely everything I had and threw it on the bed. I hadn't seen some of this stuff in years!

I separated the clothes into three piles: Keep, Out-of-Here and Maybe. I actually held every item of clothing and ran a checklist through my head: Do I still wear it? Will I ever wear it? Does it fit? If I wasn't sure about something, I tried it on. If I still wasn't sure, I took it from the Maybe pile and tried it on again. Naturally, there were some items that were no longer right for me that were still worth keeping—a gift from my mother, or a favorite sweater I might save for my niece—but I was fairly strict in my approach. I figured if I let myself chicken out on this I'd be right back where I started.

After a few hours, I emerged with three piles of clothes. I returned the Keep-ers to my pristine closet, tossed the Out-of-Heres into a bag to bring to Goodwill and boxed what I planned to give away to friends and family.

There was a great side benefit to this overhaul. It forced me to look at my clothes in basic terms. I made myself think of items I positively couldn't do without (like my beloved sweats!), and as I sorted through my stuff I realized I could be quite happy and stylish with very few essentials. After I set aside a great pair of jeans, I divided my casual clothes into six basic colors: brown, black, red, blue, white and khaki. Brown doesn't do much for me these days, unless it is a deep rich chocolate brown, so I limited myself to a pair of brown suede shoes, a belt, a bag and a pair of slacks. Black is fundamental, and here I kept a nice black blazer and trench coat, leggings, slacks, a belt, a bag, three pairs of shoes (high, low and boots), a snazzy turtleneck, one long knit skirt and one short skirt. Red made the cut with a blazer, turtleneck, and classic above-the-knee skirt; blue with a blazer and jeans. My basic whites consisted of five long-sleeved cotton, rayon and linen shirts, linen pants and a pair of Keds. In khaki, I went with two pairs of shorts, a pair of pants and a skirt. For formal wear, I made sure I had a couple of drop-dead dresses in black and red and one in dark sapphire blue, to go with my blue eyes. (Always accentuate the positive!)

From here I could build my wardrobe back up, and with this in mind I gave myself a few rules of thumb:

I. Take the time to find clothes that fit you now. Don't fall into the trap of buying for what you might look like after "the diet." Dress for your body as it is. And don't make yourself crazy for summer. I know so many women who buy small bathing suits and vow to fit themselves into them in time for their vacation. How many of those suits remain unworn, perhaps with the tags still on them? Buy something you can enjoy now, and set realistic goals. Once you accept the notion that true beauty lies within, and that there are ways to feel good about yourself that have nothing to do with a scale or a mirror, you'll likely give up the destructive diet routine. Or the ways in which you fuel yourself will become part of a total lifestyle change. You'll take better care of yourself. You'll eat healthier foods. You'll exercise more. I came to these changes when I realized I was running out of energy by the end of the day. I switched to fruit and juices in the morning, instead of my usual bagel and coffee. And I started walking at least thirty minutes at least three times a week—longer if I could find the time. As I've said before, real change takes real time. And action. And buying a too-small bathing suit is not an action with an effective result. So shop for the person you are, not the one you wish you were or hope to be.

2. Have a clear understanding of what image you want to project, and what clothes best reflect your personality.

3. Generally, keep patterns small. You want your clothes to reflect who you are, not overwhelm you.

4. Don't overaccessorize. Keep it simple. Faux pearl and cubic zirconia earrings, a pearl necklace and a brushed gold bracelet are great accessories.

5. Stay away from fabrics that love static cling! If you must wear them, do so under layers. Weighted fabrics tend to hang best on full-figured women, although knits can offer a nice exception. I like wearing a knit suit that presents my curves in a flattering way.

I never realized how important fabrics were

until I got into this business. There are several good synthetic blends available that look good on our frames. Viscose, a type of rayon, turns up in many suits, pants and blazers, and it tends not to wrinkle so it's excellent for traveling. Gabardine has a nice weight of its own, and doesn't cling like other fabrics. You can find wool gabardine and cotton gabardine blends, which give the natural fibers more versatility and flexibility.

Charmeuse feels like silk, but it's not. It's a bit heavier in weight, so it falls nicely, and it's perfect for summer. Georgette is another rayon found in a lot of formal wear, and it can work beautifully as a sheer layering tool. Among the natural fibers, silk feels soft on the skin and can be wonderful in accessories like scarves. Washable silk is not only practical, it's more versatile; it has a texture that makes it suitable for dresses, pants, jackets, you name it. And silk colors have a much longer life than they used to. Cotton is my all-time favorite; it holds its own, it breathes and it's incredibly comfortable. And you don't want to overlook crepes, and cotton and wool knits. Wool alone can be a challenge, especially those one hundred percent wool suits. For a job interview, go for a wool blend; you'll look just as beautiful, but perhaps a bit less bulky. (And you won't itch!)

What to Wear

For the longest time, large women were being sold on these ridiculous, house-dressy polyester outfits that were as uncomfortable as they were unflattering. I never owned one myself, but I've certainly modeled my share. I don't care what anyone says, there is no shape to a muumuu—probably the most unflattering garment a full-figured woman can own. And yet the department stores sell millions of muumuus each year. I don't understand it. We don't have to wear a tent to cover our frames. There are choices, women!

Comfort is essential, and I don't mean simply in relation to fit. We've all squeezed into a pair of shoes or jeans one size too small—at one time or another, for one reason or another—and yet at some point we should realize the folly in leaving the house in ill-fitting clothes. We must also consider our emotional comfort levels in deciding what to wear. Being pinched and cinched all day is no picnic, so I try to relax a bit on my own time. If you're a jeans kind of person, find a pair that fits and has some room to move in. If you need pumps, buy a pair you can wear for a stretch at the office or on the dance floor. How many of us have suffered from sore feet, and sworn never to wear "those" shoes again? The idea is to feel as good about the clothes you wear as you feel inside them. Life is too short to walk around in pain.

With pants, I like a flat panel and a slim leg,

which I find can be very flattering to someone with a thicker waist. Those of us who are wider at the bottom should look for pants with a flat-lying pleat in front, a semi-elasticized waistband, or more casual pants with a drawstring. I don't wear a lot of pants because skirts tend to look better on me, but my favorite are high-waisted wool gabardine black palazzo pants. They move beautifully and pack well.

When I see pleated skirts a red flag goes up. For me, after repeated wearings, my hips extend the width of the pleats to where they start to look like grooves. I much prefer a flat, A-line skirt. It's got a gorgeous line, and the dropped waistline is nice for an ample midsection. I also like the way the flat panel in the front doesn't add extra fullness, and if the skirt has an elastic back it can offer a nice, tailored look. I usually wear my skirts one to two inches above my knees, but not so short that I can't cross my legs without revealing too much—not a good move on an interview (unless you're Sharon Stone) or a first date (unless you're *really* interested!).

I always feel great in a classic white shirt—an excellent staple. It's not easy to find them in bigger sizes, so I tend to grab them when I see them. I'm particularly fond of those with French cuffs, which go great with an ordinary blazer and a pair of jeans. I look for an assortment of styles: a basic Oxford, tailored, frilly, long or with a tapered waist. Each can dress up a simple legging or sweater, or set off a business suit.

If you don't have any blazers in your wardrobe, think about a classic navy blue jacket. It goes with everything, and it always will. (It looks great over those white shirts!) Beyond navy, a black blazer can double for casual as well as evening wear. A lined black gabardine jacket can be worn over a simple black dress to beat the night chill in the air and maintain an elegant look. Or you can go with a nice red—not a fire-engine red, but something a bit more muted, toward a maroon.

I like a blazer that falls below my hips. There are wrap styles, and double- and single-breasted styles, and V-neck cuts. Double-breasted jackets tend to bunch up on me, so I prefer the single-breasted style. I also avoid anything with big breast pockets or substantial shoulder pads.

And speaking of substantial, I've been seeing big appliqués and large prints turning up in formal wear, but they're not to my taste. At night especially, I don't want to be seen wearing anything "fun," like bright polka dots or a loud artist's print. I like my formal clothes to be a bit more chic and simple, and somewhat sexy—not matronly. Evening wear is problematic for a lot of large-size women, but it doesn't have to be. How many times have you seen an attractive woman cloak herself in layers upon layers of clothing? Remember: Layering is an effective tool, but it's a lousy concealer.

Many women are intimidated by the prospect of layering or accessorizing as dressing tools, but you shouldn't be. Fears of winding up looking like the Michelin Man are understandable, and you certainly don't want to camouflage a terrific outfit through the wrong layering choices. But these fears shouldn't prevent you from experimenting.

Don't be afraid of not getting it right the first time. *Really* experiment. When I'm wearing a simple dress or suit or a casual outfit that I want to jazz up, I dump several potential layers—a blazer, a vest, a scarf, a shell—on my bed. Then I'll try them on with what I'm wearing: one by one, sometimes two by two. Then I check it out. Some things don't work at all. Others do, but my choice depends upon my mood or sometimes my intention. Do I want to add flair for a special party, or am I in a corporate mode? I try be be creative first, then a judge.

As I try on the different pieces, I ask myself a few questions. First, how do I look? Do the colors go together? Does the added garment seem to complete the outfit or does it compete with it? If it's not working, I'm the first to admit it. Then I'll try on something else.

Here are some general tips and guidelines to aid you in your choices:

In colder weather, turtlenecks, sweaters and vests are not only fashionable layering tools, they'll also keep you warm. However, too many thick layers will be uncomfortable. They'll inhibit movement and hide your figure, possibly giving you a frumpy look you definitely don't want. To avoid this, the trick is to identify the one layer that will be the thickest, then keep the other layers from being nearly so thick. Be sure to resist the temptation to try to obscure your figure with layer upon layer. Believe me, it won't work. And you'll only wind up feeling like that Michelin Man.

In warmer weather, simple layering is key. The materials are thinner, and there's no need to load up for warmth. Lingerie such as a bra or camisole or a bodysuit topped by a dress with buttons down the front is a beautiful choice. I often favor a "Victorian" look of a lacy tanktop under a lightweight cotton dress.

Winter or summer, I like to wear scarves two ways: draped across the back of my neck, tied once in the front and then the ends tucked into the front of my shirt, or wrapped a few times loosely around my neck, the two ends in back tucked into one of the fabric's folds.

And remember: With layering, the more you practice, the better your eye will become. If you're still feeling unsure of yourself, you can always enlist the discerning eye of a trusted friend. I've often relied on old roommates (and now my husband) for constructive criticism as I've waded through a mountain of clothes trying to choose the "right" combination.

One more word to the wise: I've found that if you buy good-quality classic basics and then some wilder, more fashion-of-the-moment accessories, you'll find you'll have a lot more outfits in your closet for a lot less money.

Speaking of keeping costs down, over the years I've found great layering items in vintage stores and local bazaars and at the Salvation Army. So check them out. You'll probably find you'll be able to go wild and still not break the bank.

Finally, about that dread layering terror: static cling! It's my worst enemy in winter when I layer with silk and polyester or when I'm on a plane. I usually have a water spritzer and a bottle of static guard handy to do battle. A couple of blasts above my head, in my pant legs or under my skirts is enough to keep it under control. I go as far as spraying a bit on my hairbrush before running it through my fine hair, too. It works. Thank God for travel-size static guard!

A lot of the designers are selling black as the primary color in formal and business attire, but I think women need a splash of something else. And yet I have the hardest time finding a good selection in other colors. Black is fine as a canvas (it can actually be quite striking when set off with some vibrant jewelry or a nice pair of heels), but big and tall women can get lost in all that darkness. If you want to turn heads you need to be creative, and mindful of your shape. I like something with a little color to it; it adds spice to the evening and helps me to feel special.

Lingerie is a hot item in large sizes. Stores can't keep up with demand, and I have to think it's connected to how we are truly beginning to feel about ourselves. Larger women are no different from their straight-size sisters in this respect. We all enjoy the sensuality of a fine undergarment (and the outcome!).

If anything, plus-size women may constitute a disproportionate percentage of the lingerie market. My clients tell me they can't keep their plus-size lingerie in the stores, on Valentine's Day especially, and I have to believe our purchases are telling.

No doubt the attraction stems in part from a desire to cut loose in private. Women want to feel especially sexy when they're with their partners. A lacey undergarment or a teddy can hopefully assist a woman's sense of her sensuality, and chase some of the feelings of inadequacy she can't help but absorb from the media's ideal of the feminine form. I know that when I put on a hot little number it changes my whole outlook.

The truth is, women of size look sensational in most lingerie styles. This is one area where size definitely counts, where more is more. Sometimes, when I stand in front of a mirror (or in front of my husband), looking voluptuous in a sexy new outfit, I'll think to myself, *Yeah, I'd like to see that girl from the jeans ad wear one of these.* I've always felt that if you've got it, you should show it off a bit, and there's no better place to put our abundant gifts on display than in the bedroom, and no better way to wrap those gifts than in some of the wonderful large-size undergarments now being sold in department and specialty stores all over the world.

So go ahead and flaunt, and leave the skinny waifs in your wake.

Another chance to highlight our sensuality is with a great swimsuit. I need a suit that stays on me when I ride the waves or swim, not something that is going to leave me naked or otherwise exposed when I leave the water. The trick is finding a suit with a good foundation built into it—one that fits your breasts and keeps them from sagging, or one that will hold you with confidence and not ride up in back. I absolutely will not buy a suit with wimpy elastic borders. High leg cuts work well for me, showing off my long legs while nipping into the look of my hips. This style draws attention to a shapely mid- to lower leg, and flatters a strong upper body.

There's something incredibly sexy about an exposed back in a bathing suit, and for most larger women that's one area they can display with aplomb. Or, in a one-piece, you might find a sheer petticoat design that flatters the line around the thigh area, and lends a gentle femininity to the look. Two-piece suits don't seem to be so popular in plus sizes, but there's no reason not to wear one. True, a lot of the designs are made with skinny, petite bodies in mind, but there are plenty of two-piece suits that would flatter a larger woman.

I wear a bikini from time to time. It took a while before I was able to relax in one on a public beach, but now I enjoy it. I am nearly alone in this, among large-size American women, but all over Europe, women wear the skimpiest bikinis on the most abundant frames. There's something refreshing about the whole approach to the human body over there.

Moving from swimwear to outerwear, I refuse to buy those enormous, shoulder-padded jackets, no matter how popular they are. They're too cumbersome for around town, especially in plus sizes. I may be a bit behind the curve on this one, but that's okay.

There's a line of "team" parkas out there that is

the latest fashion among younger women, but it's not an attractive look for someone with my build. It might be a fun, sporty look, but I prefer a warm, straight-line coat with a bit of tailoring to it. A classic woolen or camel-hair coat with a long, tapered line makes me feel statuesque and nicely highlights whatever I've got going on underneath.

Capes can look sensational on all women. They're one of the few items of clothing we can all wear with flair, so we might as well take advantage of them. With capes, the bigger you are, the less it matters. On a cool evening, there's no sharper accent to your outfit than a long, elegant cape—maybe even with a hood. It lends a wonderful, willowy kind of look to your ensemble, and spotlights your size in a beautiful way.

Coats and capes are perhaps the one exception to my practice of buying things I can enjoy today. Here I shop for tomorrow, out of season. Styles don't change all that much from one year to the next. The close-out savings can be substantial, particularly in a high-end style with some tailoring to it.

Shopping for shoes is another one of my dreaded activities. Large women tend to have large feet (if we didn't, we'd topple right over!), but there isn't exactly a large, stylish selection to accommodate us. There are a few national chains that stock a good variety of widths and lengths. (You'll find a list of stores and catalogues in the appendix at the back of this book.) I look for comfort first, and settle for the rest. A shoe with a strong arch support is essential for me—as I suspect it is for a lot of you. I also want something that doesn't throw me forward toward my toe. High, high heels are tough, but an inch or so lends a nice lift to the calf, and elongates the leg.

Ruby red slippers are out. In shoes, I'm leery of anything too loud, which could call too much attention to one of my least attractive features. Neutral tones like tan, black and brown are a safer choice. For casual wear, a white canvas sneaker can be just right with a pair of jeans. Sneakers are fine for an active outing, but for an informal get-together, I prefer a basic flat, or an espadrille. Boots offer another casual option, and a wider range of choices. Some of the men's styles look great on larger women; in cowboy boots especially, the styles are close enough that even a real cowboy won't know the difference.

Just as true beauty comes from within, so too does style. The hottest outfit in the world is nothing on a lifeless frame, whereas the simplest outfit can be everything when worn with the right attitude. Don't just take my word for it. Experiment, and develop a style all your own. And remember: Your clothes should flatter you, not represent you; you represent yourself.

15

Taking Charge

Among the 1996 finalists for the prestigious Westinghouse science scholarships awarded to the nation's top high-school students was a young woman from Lawrence, New York, named Juliette Taska, and she was honored for the simple way she located one of the root ills of our diet-obsessed society. She rates a mention here for the same.

Juliette, a cross-country and track athlete, noticed a brief article in a back issue of *Runner's World* magazine, spotlighting a straightforward nutritional study being conducted at Macalester College in St.

Paul, Minnesota. A professor there was doing some interesting work seeking a correlation between advertising and dieting, on the theory that certain messages actually encouraged certain kinds of people to eat.

For a long time, Juliette and her friends had been talking about crash diets—about why they never seemed to work, about how the diet companies set impossible standards, about how certain people were never able to control what they ate—and in this small item she hit upon a big idea: Why not pull together a group of her classmates and mirror the Macalester study in her own school?

"I'd always thought that diet commercials make us want to eat more, not less," she explained, after her findings were reported in local newspapers, "and this seemed a good way to find out if it was true."

Juliette assembled ninety of her female classmates, concocted a cover story that she was studying appetites of young women at various points in their menstrual cycles, and attempted to prove her point. She separated her friends into two groups, invited each to separate screenings of the tearjerkingest Hollywood movie she could find (the four-hankie classic *Terms of Endearment*), and set out measured amounts of M&Ms and salted peanuts in easy reach of every viewer. The groups were mixed according to age and to ethnic and economic backgrounds. Before the screenings, Juliette spliced one movie tape with body-image commercials for products like shampoo and makeup, and the other with neutral advertisements promoting trucks and overnight delivery services. She also had participants fill out questionnaires, indicating whether or not they were prone to dieting.

The idea, she said, was to see if likely dieters assaulted with commercials featuring models and beauty-care products would snack more frequently than likely dieters confronted with neutral messages, and if non-dieters were prone to the same impulses.

"The movie was important because it was a strong emotional distraction," Juliette said. "It put everyone in a susceptible state. This way, the focus was on what was happening to Debra Winger, and not on the commercials, and hopefully not on the eating. I wanted to see what everyone ate when they weren't thinking about it, when their minds were on something else."

What Juliette found didn't exactly surprise her, but it did confirm some of her hunches. The dieters in the body-image commercial group ate twice as much as the dieters in the control group. Twice as much! And keep in mind, these "body-image" commercials weren't directly promoting specific diets or diet products; what they were selling, really, was an outward ideal, a way of meeting the world with your best face forward, yet the message triggered some kind of craving among the more vulnerable students in the study.

"I was expecting the result," Juliette reflected later. "That's basically what they found in the original study. But what I still don't get is the why. Why does the sight of a super-thin model make us reach for the candy? Why does even thinking about our hair or our nail polish make us hungry? Maybe it's the psychological intimidation factor. You know, maybe we start to think, Why am I kidding myself? I see all these beautiful people on television and in magazines and it's impossible for me to look like that so I might as well eat. What this tells us is that the commercials themselves change a person's mood and make them want to eat more. That's a dangerous thing."

With her friends at school, Juliette said she stands mostly alone. At five feet tall, and one hundred pounds, with a strong, athletic build, she's not faced with the same issues as other teenage girls. Her active workout schedule keeps her from doing battle on the scales. "Around here, skinny is beautiful," she admitted, "just like anyplace else, but it would be great if health and fitness were just as important. To a lot of kids, it's how you look that counts, not how you feel. What they don't realize is that the typical healthy person actually is beautiful."

No, Juliette, they don't. And it's not just high-school students who don't get the message. We're all a little messed up on this one, caught in a bad place at a bad time. Yes, we're defenseless against all sorts of media messages; yes, we've lost sight of where we've been in terms of what we once held as beautiful; yes, we want instant gratification; and yes, we're impatient for trends to turn back in our favor. We look at the out-of-date height-to-weight recommendations in our doctors' offices or on life insurance charts and see only the low end. Statistics don't lie, but they don't always tell the whole truth. If the numbers say we should weigh between one hundred ten and one hundred thirty pounds, most women will shoot for one hundred ten, when in fact they might have a body that takes them naturally to the other end of the range. We've forgotten that it's a *range* of weight we're talking about. We've conditioned ourselves to believe that less is more, when more can be exactly right.

Advertisers have done such a good job with their seduction and persuasion techniques that women buy products because they *need* to, not because they want to. Do we believe everything we're told, and sold? Stop and ask yourself what is going on here, and you might find some of the answers within yourself. Let's put some of the responsibility back into our own hands. I'm not one to talk. I'm always in search of the perfect moisturizer; I've tried at least fifty brands. Pathetic? I think so. Whenever I thought I'd found the perfect one, I'd be enticed by the next commercial to try another.

I can't imagine a period when first impressions have been more important than they are right now. Our lives are so busy, so programmed, that we haven't left ourselves any time for missteps. We don't trust ourselves to grow on someone, or them to grow on us. We want what we want as soon as we want it. We're convinced that if we hope to live/work/play/love a certain way, we need to do it in a certain kind of body. We need to do this with our face, and this with our boobs and this with our thighs. If we don't, we'll never be happy. We've gotten to where we'll do everything but be ourselves. We live on everybody's terms but our own.

I think about these things and worry we'll be mired in this mode for the next while, but I believe we can find our way out in little steps. Let's start small. If we work to make a difference in our own lives, if we *try*, we'll eventually shake some sense into the collective middle. We need only look to each other for inspiration.

For all the strides we've made in the last several years, we still live in a culture where larger women keep mostly to themselves. It's not necessarily our own doing, but it's a done deal just the same. I travel a lot for my modeling jobs, and I notice very few businesswomen larger than a size ten or twelve. It never struck me as strange until I sat down to write this book, when I realized I saw hundreds of women each day, coming in and out of our major airports, and almost all of them are not over a size fourteen. They're dressed to the teeth, but they're under size twelve. I always hear stories of larger women having great telephone personalities, being more comfortable working behind the scenes. What a load! How many people do you know wouldn't be comfortable with a great job, and the chance to travel, to contribute at the front lines of a going concern? We have great telephone personalities because that's all most employers want from us.

What does it say about us as a society that we see a need to hide our "imperfections"? You'd never see a bald-headed man being passed over for a power position in his firm. (Okay, so he might wear a toupee, but that's another story.) A guy with a beer belly isn't kept from advancing. Granted, appearances play a huge part in American business, I understand that, but there's a clear double standard. Men can look however they want, but women need to fit the prototype.

In Germany, for example, appearances also matter, but over there it's all about great shoes, great suits, excellent color schemes, the finest materials. Men and women are judged, or not judged, equally. I've seen German women—size sixteen, eighteen, twenty—walking around in the same suits as their slimmer colleagues. And they look classy. They're in positions of power and they fit right in.

In Italy, the men are very expressive with their admiration. Nowhere else have I had the positive, nonabusive attention I get when I'm in Florence, where a woman is seen as a tremendous asset; the more you have, the more you have to give. I don't see this as a backlash to the changing trends, but an indication that Italian men know exactly what they want. They love us in all our shapes! *Grazie!*

I sometimes think the pendulum has swung to where our bodies are once again judged along class lines in American society, only now we delineate class in a new way. Now it's all about power and control. Now if you eat, and gain weight, it somehow means you're weak, you have no willpower, no self-control.

The more we restrain ourselves, the more in charge we're supposed to be. I believe it's all tied in to some pretty messed-up notions of success. The beautiful people are supposed to have money, right? If you're thin, you've got power; if you've got power, you've got money; if you've got money, you've found happiness. Somehow, that's how it equates. New York, Chicago, Atlanta, Miami, Los Angeles . . . it's always the same thing. It's ridiculous, but I see it everywhere, among our young people especially. We seem to want the appearance of being in control, without actually being in control of anything. We seem to want to restrain ourselves just for the sake of restraining ourselves, just to show the world that we can.

If we don't do something about it soon, we'll remain helpless against it.

*P*ause

The good news about self-acceptance is that you can work on it whenever you want to—all the time, if you like! After all, you're always available to yourself.

Society may seem like a tougher nut to crack. It is. And it's often harder to gauge changes happening at such a wide level. Every now and then we'll get hints and signposts that the world is coming our way. I took my inclusion in *People* magazine's "The 50 Most Beautiful People in the World" as such a sign. But even then it's hard to tell the difference between an anomaly and a trend. We need to continue to focus on our efforts and look for those signs. Mainly, we need to continue our efforts. The results, for the most part, will be tough to measure. So we can't let ourselves get discouraged by what may seem to be a lack of change. Just when we think things aren't changing at all, they may be changing the most.

So how can we, on an individual basis, change the world? We can start by being more demanding consumers.

That I am a model at all signals the fact that clothing manufacturers and retail stores are finally wising up to the fact that plus-size women constitute sixty percent of their market. They aren't courting our business because they think it's the right thing to do; they're doing it because it's the sensible thing to do. They're courting our business because they want our business. Our business is valuable. Just keep that in mind every time you make any financial transaction, be it for goods or services.

Since our business is valuable, retailers should be interested to know what we want. And even if they don't seem to be at first, we need to keep telling them. Every time you go shopping and you can't find decent or fashionable clothes in your size, you should let the retailers know that they are missing out on your business because of their inability to provide the items you desire. Don't just mutter your gripe to a sales clerk. Ask to speak to a manager. Better yet, a buyer. Depending on the store, the manager or buyer really might not know that sixty percent of American women are size twelve or higher. So be polite, but make your case clear. Think of your role as that of an educator. You want clothes that fit you. Fashionable clothes in decent fabrics. The same as any size-ten woman would want. You are a consumer, you have money, and you are willing to pay. And there are a lot more of you out there.

We will be heard only if we are willing to stand up for ourselves. I know it's difficult. It's insisting on our rights by insisting on the very features that make us most anxious about ourselves. But if we don't stand up for ourselves, who will? And if we stand up together, just think how powerful our voices can be.

This willingness to be heard also applies to a willingness to be seen. I know many of us are shy about going to health clubs. All those skinny, muscular bodies decked out in the latest Lycra blends. It's not fun feeling like the Michelin tire man among all those hard bodies, but we need to be brave. *Everyone* feels insecure from time to time. Wear clothes that are comfortable, and show up. Most clubs have fitness specialists available for help designing programs that are right for club members. Don't be shy about asking one to help develop a program for you. (It is also recommended that you consult a physician before embarking on any exercise program.)

Maybe you won't be running seven miles at a fast clip or doing the StairMaster for an hour and a half, but there is an appropriate starting point for everyone. Don't be shy about asking for help finding yours. Ask to speak to a trainer. Be honest about where you are with respect to physical fitness. Ask for help in designing an aerobic program that is right for you. Then follow through on that program.

After you've tried it a few times, talk to the

trainer again. Many programs need fine-tuning. And as you get fitter, you may want to beef up your program. Again, consult that trainer. That's what they're there for. And if they're like the trainers I know, they like nothing better than working with an interested health-club member who will listen to what they have to say.

I know you'll feel anxious. I know you may feel like you're sticking out. All I can say is, take a deep breath and get over it. No one is going to stick up for your rights for you. No one can assert yourself in these situations but you. If you don't start somewhere, you can't progress. And once you do get over it, once you get over that first stumbling block and get started, you'll find that showing up becomes easier and easier every time.

Travel is another area that is problematic for many of us. All those narrow seats on planes, trains and buses. When I'm flying, I always ask for an aisle seat. My travel agent knows my preference and just automatically books it for me. I feel like I have more room on the aisle, and I don't have to climb over people to get out of my seat. Depending on how crowded a plane is, you can also ask to move to a seat that has an empty one by it. Then you can lift the armrest between the two seats and get more room.

Again, this is one of those situations where you're going to have to take the initiative. You're going to have to ask for yourself. Even if a stewardess thinks of moving you so you can have more room, she may not offer you the other seat for fear of offending you. So you have to be the one to ask.

Whenever you're dealing with any of these people—the store manager or buyer, the health-club trainer, the stewardess—remind yourself that you'll set the tone for the conversation. You're initiating that conversation. The person to whom you are speaking will pick up the tone from you. So if you're giving yourself a pep talk in advance of speaking to them, remind yourself that you are completely within your rights. Your request is worthy of consideration. You are worthy. Try not to let yourself be flustered or embarrassed. Do not apologize; you are not in the wrong! State your request or question calmly. Look the person in the eye, but do not challenge them. If you are complaining about something, by your tone and manner let the person to whom you are speaking know that you are not holding them to blame. If they seem to think you are blaming them, tell them explicitly that you are not. You are simply expressing your complaint/request to them as

Emme

representatives of the store/health club/airline.

You may find a warmer reception than you anticipated. If the clothing business is a sign of the times, I think we'll be seeing more retailers, manufacturers and service providers catering to our needs and cultivating our business. For our part, we need to express ourselves. We need to be willing to stand up to be counted if we want to be heard.

16

Developing a Personal Style

Avery successful strategy in aiding us to accept our bodies is to develop a personal style. What works for the waif probably won't work for us. You might look for a fashion model whose body image approximates yours, but she may not be out there—at least not yet. So until we see more people in the media who look like us, we'll have to rely on our own creativity. There's no excuse for not being original! Don't think of it as a challenge so much as an opportunity.

For starters—and to free you up—let me give you

one fabulously outrageous example of a woman who grew so tired of the paucity of fashions and role models available to plus-size women that she went out and crafted her own.

Joan is an antiques dealer from northern California. A size twenty-two, she'd given up on dieting. She felt that she didn't have the motivation to exercise. She didn't like the way she looked or the way she carried herself, but she was resigned to her body. So one morning she woke up and decided to challenge everyone's expectations of what she should look like. To do it, she decided to go against the grain. So she shaved her head, bought some blue and orange lipstick and some shockingly loud jewelry and tossed out her old wardrobe in favor of flowing capes and outlandish haberdashery. She'll be the first to admit there was something Halloweenish in her approach, but when she stepped out into the world, no one was likely to forget her.

"People looked at me differently right away," Joan recalls. "It was like this tremendous awakening. My whole life, I'd worn these ridiculous muumuu things. I was always kind of shrinking into a corner, but I just had had enough. I don't know what it was that set me off, but something did. I weighed two hundred and forty pounds, and believe me it's tough to hide that kind of body, but somehow I managed, and people were pretty compliant in letting me get away with it.

"But I reached the point where I needed to step out and do something. I needed to call attention to myself. I'd lived in constant fear of being noticed, but that's exactly what I needed. I needed to dress *up*. I needed to get out. I needed to just be. If I didn't, I'd go crazy in the head, so I went a little crazy with my clothes and makeup. I don't have a problem with that. Hey, it's not all that different from some of these ridiculous outfits you see on the runways in Paris. Those girls just want to turn heads, too. I can't wear those styles, but I can develop my own."

These days, Joan figures she's turned so many heads her neighbors must have chronic whiplash. "It's almost like a game to me now," she admits, "to try and be a little more shocking, a little more out there. I let myself be intimidated for so long, I figured it was time for me to do the intimidating. I don't care if people are uncomfortable around me. I truly don't. Better that than me being uncomfortable around them. Once, I actually went to a dealers' convention wearing an eye patch. Just to shake things up a little. And these people all knew me. They knew I had no trouble with my eyes, but no one thought to ask if I was okay or anything. I thought that was just great. 'Oh, you know, that's just Joan.'"

Joan's choices may be far too extreme for your taste, but think of her as somewhere way out there in the limitless range of possibilities. Be encouraged. Feel liberated. Be bold. Don't be afraid to experiment until you find a style that works for you.

Don't be afraid to be consistent, either. If you find a particular style of blouse that fits and works well for you, why not buy it in several available shades? The same is true of pants and skirts. If you're concerned about the monotony, there's certainly a lot you can do in the way of accessorizing that will enhance your style.

Don't be afraid to buck fashion trends with respect to your clothes. If tight-fitting tops with a midriff revealed are all the rage, don't feel obliged to jump on the bandwagon—unless you're game for it. Feel free to decide.

You can always "go wild" with a single outfit or article of clothing. What may seem harder to experiment with is your hair. If you've really found the style that works for you, by all means stick with it. But many women may wear their hair a certain way just because that's the way they've always worn it.

If you think you might be overdue for a change, go to a hairdresser you trust. Make an appointment just to talk to your stylist. Forget about photos of hairstyles you like. What looks good in a photo probably won't be a match for you in terms of your type of hair and your face shape. Discuss some possibilities with your stylist, then go mull it over. A new hairstyle may be just the change you're looking for.

I just don't recommend change for change's sake. I like weighing the options. But then, maybe that's part of my personal style. It may not be part of yours!

17

Finding Your Comfort Zone

To understand how we are sometimes made to feel by the society in which we live, we must make an effort to understand the world around us and to take responsibility for our place within it. And we must accept that there are ebbs and flows to our societal values: What's in today is out tomorrow. There's a pendulum at work here, and we can't sit and wait for it to swing back before we start feeling better about ourselves. We have to kind of push things along a little.

Consider: The path between Twiggy and Kate Moss has not exactly been a straight one, but it's taken us to the same place. Here we are. Again. (And so soon!) Along the way, we briefly made room for the all-American fresh-faced blonde, who told us it was okay to be a little fleshier, a little big in the chest. Remember when cleavage was in? And full-wattage smiles? For a short time, beginning in the late 1970s, Cheryl Ladd, Farrah Fawcett and Christie Brinkley all offered a more vibrant lifestyle choice, but the pendulum has swung back to the impossible über-waif model.

This troubles me. Perhaps it troubles you. We can't all be the flavor of the month, every month. If we could, we'd miss out on all those fun emotions like envy and frustration and grudging resentment. We wouldn't know what it is to feel guilty about what we eat, or shame at how we look. We need to have something to shoot for, something to miss out on, something to beat ourselves up about. It keeps things interesting.

Think about the messages we are assaulted with on a daily basis—in magazines, on television, at the multiplex, on the local news. I'm not just talking about the advertisements, although they play a big part of it, but the overall picture. What hits home for way too many of us is that money can buy absolutely anything, even emotional satisfaction. (Excuse me, but didn't the Beatles sing a different tune?)

Are we being supported or persuaded to be who we want to be? Are we encouraged to live rich, fulfilling lives with depth and balance? I don't think so. The way I see it, our world is all about who can make the biggest buck on insignificant products that can't possibly deliver the happiness they promise. We are constantly being told that if we buy this juicer or that tummy exerciser we will feel better, look better, become whole. Does that make sense? When did our mass consumption replace the basic warmth and security of positive human relationships in solving our problems? Have we distanced ourselves from our feelings to the point where we no longer communicate when we need love, respect or a listening ear? For that matter, do we really believe that material things are the answer? Some purchases may yield a short-term boost, but that's about where it ends. Yes, certain goodies do make me happy, to a certain extent, but there is a point at which I look around at all my purchases and wonder what in the world I was thinking.

Let's face it, the only one who can make a substantial difference in your life is you. That's what it comes down to. Nothing you could possibly buy from a catalogue or late-night infomercial could ever do as much for you as you can do for yourself. Even a motivational book such as this one is only a starting point for the hard (but positive!) work that lies ahead. I know this from experience. Throughout my life, whenever I needed a lift, I spent money on every cure-all I could find, even when I didn't have the money to spend, when what I truly needed was a hug, a friend or a spiritual connection. My overeating during these times reflected a real lack of control, of not being able to fulfill my needs on the very deepest emotional levels. My actions make sense to me now, but it was hell at the time, and it was only after I'd developed a nurturing network of friends that I was able to find the support I needed to change my bad habits. It was kind of like training a dog, the way I retrained myself. I learned not to tear myself down, not to find fault with myself for not being perfect.

The key to my personal salvation was reaching out—not just to other people, but also reaching outside myself to place the validation I needed in the world around me. My support group of friends, mentors and my patient and ever-loving husband Phil helped me immensely, but I was the one who finally got mad enough to stand up for myself. I'd had enough. I wouldn't put myself down anymore. There were enough people out there waiting to do it for me, but the real revelation was that there were a great many more who were suffering what I was suffering. I finally got it: If you don't feel deserving of your place in the community, then you will never truly belong. It took wanting to make others feel better about themselves to make me feel better. It took belonging to finally belong. It took listening to other women talk about their weight problems, their low self-esteem, their negative body images to get me to understand my own, and to move on.

I wasn't alone, and neither are you, and I sincerely hope the message clicks. Please know that the more I reached outside myself, the more I saw myself as I truly was. Why is it that we tend to push each other away? Are we afraid of being judged and deemed unworthy? Are we conditioned to think that our values must be determined by the latest trends? What's clear is that we all need a safe haven, a place to be real, with each other and with ourselves. It's a shame that more of us can't lean on others with similar experiences to see us through the bad times, but it doesn't have to be that way. Let's take things back to how they were, before the electronic age diluted our ability to interact with each other. Let's give our old ways of doing things another try. Start small: There are probably a dozen people in your neighborhood looking for a walking buddy or a running partner each morning. Seek each other out. Your family might need a family-fitness jump start. Help each other out. Talk to each other. You'll be amazed at the results.

Recently, Phil and I lunched at an Italian restaurant in the mall next to our home. We sat down near a table of four women, and they were rattling on about what their new exercise equipment would do to their misshapen body parts. Their whole meal was devoted to calories consumed, hours spent exercising and what new products they were thinking of buying. Our eavesdropping set the tone for the entire day. Later, on a checkout line, we heard one woman boasting to her friend how much weight she had lost on a "fabulous" new diet. And still later, in a dress shop, I watched a forty-something woman struggle into an outfit meant for someone half her age, and half her size.

What was going on in that shopping mall was little different from what goes on every day in every corner of this country. We have become so addicted to the pursuit of bodily perfection that we've seemed to trade in our uniqueness in the bargain. Who's perfect, anyway? Who is setting the standards? (And why are we letting them?) If it were possible to attain the "perfect" body, what would we work on next?

I don't mean to suggest that physical self-improvement is a bad thing. In fact, I encourage it, but I encourage it as part of the package and not as the whole deal. Once we define ourselves by our appearance, we've lost the essence of who we are. Mind, body and spirit. Sure, some of us can achieve a perfect, Barbielike figure, but in doing so at the expense of everything else, we lose the unique individual we are meant to be.

And here's another thing: I take issue with many women who are convinced they are the prisoners of a slow metabolism or a "set point." According to the set-point theory, our bodies naturally hover around a certain weight—a weight it's very tough to get below. The problem with the slow metabolism and set-point theories is that, if you subscribe to them, you can't be at fault. Your weight becomes a fait accompli, determined by nature, possibly genes, probably set for you since birth. I absolutely acknowledge that many overweight people suffer from a slow metabolism. My problem with this and the set-point theory is that they are too deterministic. And they remove that aspect of personal responsibility. How many women, I wonder, would really like to adopt a healthier diet or exercise program but they shy away from doing so because they have accepted that they have a slow metabolism or a set point? How many women are hovering well above what would be a healthy weight for them because they have bought into one of these deterministic theories?

I tend to reject any excuse that lets us off the hook too easily. To me, they're actually *un*-empowering and self-defeating. It takes a lot of strength to change the way we feel about ourselves. It's hard—and harder still because we are expected to have the same ideal. Worse, we expect it of ourselves. None of our agony and agonizing about body image transpires without our doing. That's the good news and the bad news. Bad because it's troubling that we torture ourselves needlessly yet willingly, good because the key to our ultimate liberation has been in our hands all along.

To set the right pendulum, we must first understand that we're laboring under an ironic ideal. The waifish cover girl, the sculpted body-builder, the silicon-enhanced swimsuit model, the toned athlete, the larger-than-life matinee idol . . . the objects of our perfection are themselves imperfect, which in some ways leaves the rest of us mimicking a paragon that doesn't even exist.

Get real: No one looks so photographically correct without tremendous effort—and considerable retouching! The straight-size models I hang out with are always obsessing about their weight, or starving themselves, or spending time down at the gym. A lot of male models I know won't eat for two days before a shoot, in order to achieve the desired definition in their upper body. Hollywood stars have so much work to do on their bodies in order to shine on the big screen that they hire personal trainers to do the work for them. It's such a completely unnatural way to be, and yet we've allowed these models to set our standard. This is what we aspire to, and we should have our heads examined.

What we need, therefore, is to create a place in which we might feel good about ourselves. We need to find a reasonable comfort zone. We need to set ourselves up to succeed, and not to fail.

Just how do we accomplish this? Well, we get there by degrees. Instead of seizing on one hot model or actress as an iconographic ideal, why can't we think in categories? Let's have a hot ectomorphic model, a hot endomorphic model and a hot mesomorphic model. For every Uma Thurman, let there be a Rosie O'Donnell; for every Mel Gibson, a John Goodman. Let's take in a mix of images, focus on the ones that fit, and file the rest away. If you're a big-boned, full-figured woman, there's no point in emulating a skinny little thing in a jeans ad. If you ain't got it, you ain't got it. After all, she doesn't have what you have, either.

What we need is to be realistic about the bodies

into which we were born, and work with what we've got. Unfortunately, it's not enough to strike a pragmatic pose and cast it in bronze. Try clay instead. We need to be a bit flexible on this one. The human body is not a fixed instrument. A woman's body goes through enormous changes, as a matter of course, and with each change comes a corresponding change in our metabolism. If it's not one thing, it's another. Adolescence, post-adolescence, pregnancy, lactation, pre-menopause, menopause . . . it's almost like we're forced to reinvent ourselves every seven years or so, so maybe what we need are a series of ten-year plans for looking our best.

Why is it so much easier for American men to grow old, to go gray, to develop abdominal obesity? We women have got this whole assortment of normal physiological and hormonal changes that are completely out of our control. It's a constant battle. On the one hand, we want these changes to happen; if they didn't, we'd be dead. But on the other, we've allowed ourselves to be intimidated by the status quo. We want to be how we were, not how we are. We're being asked to accept a new body every decade, to take on a new image, and we must remain open to that. We must adapt. Our body metabolism slows with age, so if we try to get through our adulthoods with the same levels of exercise relative to food intake we will naturally gain weight. The routine we followed at age twenty will yield extra pounds at age forty.

Change happens, so let's just deal with it.

Commerce happens, too, and we need designers and department stores willing to stretch the parameters of their business to include the majority of American women. It's amazing to me that the fashion industry chooses to serve only a narrow segment of the population. I don't mean to belabor the point, but the numbers offer a pretty good case. If sixty percent of us are a size twelve or larger, it makes good business sense to offer us the same styles and selections as the more streamlined woman. We're an untapped market. Tap us. Please. I promise you we'll answer back. And the same goes for women on the petite end of the range; they have as much trouble buying twos and fours off the rack as we do buying our sizes.

Let everyone walk the same cutting edge, and let us do it in shoes that fit *and* have some style to them.

Of course, we need a lot more than accoutrements to rebuild our values. We need a society-wide attitude adjustment. We need the folks who design airplanes and buses and commuter trains to be a bit more accommodating of larger-size people. We need theaters to offer more comfortable (and more forgiving) seating. We need the moguls behind our movies and magazines to celebrate a variety of images. We need to place our own self-esteem ahead of the regard we hold for people we'll never even meet. We need to teach that self-esteem to our children. We need to get them starting to think about what they put into their mouths. We also need to tell them it's okay to have an appetite, and that it's okay to make room in that appetite for things like spare ribs and ice cream and a second slice of pizza. We've let weight become the issue when what we need is to make health the priority. And family. And friends. And work. And play. We need to find ways to validate ourselves away from our bodies; we all have things to offer that have nothing to do with the way we look, so let's place our emphasis there. I'm not saying we should let ourselves go and eat with no concern for our health, but a healthy attitude is as important as anything else.

Let's also move away from this idea that we have to be one hundred percent perfect, one hundred percent of the time. How ridiculous is that? There are no such things as airbrushes in real life, so perfection is a doomed goal. The true key is balance. If you eat too much one night, go easy the next, but don't deny yourself the pleasure of a delicious meal. Discover your "reasonable weight" and do your best to stick to it. And don't be unreasonable about your doctor's recommended weight ranges. Find happiness in the middle range, or at the high end. It's foolish to think you can diet your way down to a weight you've never before achieved as an adult; if you didn't weigh one hundred twenty pounds in college, you can't expect to weigh one hundred twenty pounds at your daughter's graduation.

And finally, while we're on the subject of dieting, let's work to lose our attachment to the term. I wrote earlier that the word *fat* will be banned from my household when I have children, and I intend to show *diet* the same door. For so many of us, the word is tied up with issues of failure, inadequacy and disappointment. We talk about it as if it's some sort of mode we're entering into, as something that defines us; we've let *dieting* become a euphemism for *not eating*, and as such it no longer serves its purpose. We should do ourselves a favor and approach the process from a different angle. I don't see why we even need to slap a label on it; after all, we're not dieting so much as altering our eating habits, so let's not pay it any more notice than it deserves.

We can be anything we want, as long as we set our own standards, and our own terms. We just need to help each other, and ourselves.

Pause

Imagine you find a penny by the side of the road, heads up. You're in the middle of nowhere, and the coin has been assaulted for years by the elements. It's all dirty and rusted and oxidized; poor Abe is rubbed away to a blur; it's no more a penny than a slug.

At first, you think it's not worth the trouble, but you stoop to pick it up and an amazing thing happens. You flip it to its tail side and find a brilliant copper sheen, which reflects the morning sun like the day it was minted.

Okay, so what does this all mean? Well, for me, it serves as a reminder that we've all got our brilliant copper sheens, just waiting to be turned over. This happened to me once, and this is where it took me; whatever you've done with your life, whatever you haven't done, you can always turn things over and start fresh. Every single day, we can make our lives brand new. We can be the best we can be. Don't let the dirty, rusty and oxidized parts weigh you down. Know that if you lift yourself up and dust yourself off, you'll find a better you underneath. (Really!)

Know that with time comes understanding, and that with understanding comes forgiveness, and that with forgiveness comes strength.

Know that there are parts of your personality just waiting to be discovered.

Know that if you leave things to sit they'll only get worse.

Know that if you pick yourself up and clean yourself up you can turn things around.

18

It Has to Do

It has to do with a lot of things, I realize now. It has to do with knowing the person you've been, the person you are, the person you want to become. It has to do with keeping yourself in perspective.

It has to do with recognizing what you want and knowing how to get it.

It has to do with believing in yourself.

It has to do with faith and trust—faith in something or someone bigger than you are; trust in the belief that anything is possible.

It has to do with love.

It has to do with setting realistic goals, and working your ass off to meet them. (Someone once told me it has to do also with setting unrealistic goals, just to give yourself something to shoot for.)

It has to do with finding positive impressions on which to build.

It has to do with looking beyond your "trouble" spots and discovering aspects of character or physical traits to cherish and admire. The mirror doesn't lie. Embrace the parts of your body and personality that make you feel good. And don't reject the rest of the package. Accept it; work on it; learn from it. It's part of who you are, and who you will always be.

It has to do with tolerance. See yourself as you wish to be seen; see others as they wish to be seen; help the rest of us to see the difference.

It has to do with kindness. Be aggressively kind and it will find you on the rebound.

It has to do with folly. Don't be afraid to cut loose, have fun, defy convention. Grin and bear it. Good things come to those who smile—including laugh lines! It's better than the alternative, and there are way too many serious people in this world.

It has to do with perseverance. If something's not working, press on.

It has to do with overcoming your past, anticipating your future and sidestepping the obstacles in between. Broken homes, broken hearts and broken dreams will all set you back, that's for sure. But they won't knock you out unless you let them. Watch your back and watch your step, but keep your eyes on the path ahead.

It has to do with responsibility. If every action has an equal and opposite reaction, let's just strap ourselves in and face the consequences. Make your own choices knowing that if you overindulge in one area you'll need to compensate in another. To win one battle you'll likely have to lose another. Recognize the back and forth, and thrive in the middle.

It has to do with rejecting some of our more commonly held notions of beauty in favor of the ones that make sense. With two kids and two jobs it's impossible to make a fashion statement every time you leave the house. Accept that it's probably foolish to try. But to the one who loves you, you will always look like a page out of the Victoria's Secret catalogue. Keep in mind that you can still turn the right heads when it matters most.

It has to do with living at the edges of opportunity, and knowing when to look over the side.

It has to do with resisting the impulse to fit the mold. There is only one Claudia Schiffer, and there is only one you. Do you need to eat healthy? You bet. Do you need to keep fit? Absolutely. But stay with the program and applaud your raw materials. Create your own model. Let others follow in your path.

It has to do with inspiration. We find our impulses in the unlikeliest places: in my date book ("That which doesn't kill us only makes us stronger"); on a friend's refrigerator ("Eat, or be eaten"); on a New Hampshire license plate, mounted on the wall of another friend's office ("Live free or die").

It has to do with keeping one foot in reality and the other in fantasy.

It has to do with accepting change. As the world turns, so do we, for good or ill. No, you won't be fitting into your high-school cheerleading outfit any time soon. So what? There's probably a hot number at the boutique downtown that will look just great on you, and serve the same purpose. (Besides, who wants to look at a grown woman dressed like a cheerleader?)

It has to do with wanting something so badly you can taste it. I hate to fall back on tired eating metaphors, but if you mean to make something happen, you must visualize it and sensualize it and actualize it. Taste. Imagine. Know. And there it will be.

It has to do with understanding what works, and what doesn't. Shadow your flaws, showcase your gifts and give it your best shot.

It has to do with reason. Think it through.

It has to do with balance. Adjust your levels of work and play; diet and exercise; rest and motion. Find the mix that leaves you stable, and running smoothly. Counter each craziness with a moment of sanity.

It has to do with forgiveness. We all mess up, in big ways and small, so let's not kill each other over the past. What's the point? Grant full pardons, but always remember the transgression. Let it teach you something. And pass on what you've learned.

It has to do with respect. For yourself. For others. For new ideas.

It has to do with peace. I'm not talking about global peace, or racial peace, or peace among neighbors—good things, all! Inner peace is what counts. Everything falls from here.

It has to do with living. It's not enough to go through the motions. Give yourself over to life and see what happens.

It has to do. Period.

Dreams have a habit of coming true.
All you have to do is get in the habit of dreaming.

Recommended Reading

I wanted to share some books that have helped me get through some rough spots and see things in a variety of perspectives. I hope the next book you choose will touch you and take you on another journey to understanding more about you and your world. Enjoy!

1. *American Beauty*, Lois W. Banner (New York: Alfred A. Knopf, 1993)

2. *The Beauty Myth*, Naomi Wolf (New York: William Morrow, 1991)

3. *When Women Stop Hating Their Bodies: Freeing Yourself from Food and Weight Obsession* (New York: Random House, 1995) and *Overcoming Overeating: Living Free in a World of Food*

(Reading, MA: Addison-Wesley, 1985), Jane R. Hirschmann and Carol H. Munter

4. *Intuitive Eating,* Elise Resch, M.S., R.D., and Evelyn Tribole, M.S., R.D. (New York: St. Martin's Press, 1995)

5. *Appearance Obsession: Learning to Love the Way You Look,* Joni E. Johnston, Psy.D. (Deerfield Beach, FL: Health Communications, Inc., 1994)

6. *Fat Is a Feminist Issue: The Anti-Diet Guide to Permanent Weight Loss,* Susie Orbach (New York: Paddington Press, 1978)

7. *A Woman's Worth* (New York: Random House, 1993) and *A Return to Love: Reflections on the Principles of a Course in Miracles* (New York: HarperCollins, 1992), Marianne Williamson

8. *Self-Esteem Comes in All Sizes,* Carol A. Johnson (New York: Doubleday, 1995)

9. *Father Hunger,* Margo Maine, Ph.D. (Carlsbad, CA: Gurze Design and Book, 1991)

10. *When Words Hurt: How to Keep Criticism from Undermining Your Self-Esteem,* Mary Lynne Heldmann (Chicago: New Chapter Press, 1988)

11. *Fat Is a Family Affair,* Judi Hollis, Ph.D. (Center City, MN: Hazelden, 1985)

12. *Feeding the Hungry Heart: The Experience of Compulsive Eating* (Indianapolis, IN: Bobbs-Merrill, 1982) and *When Food Is Love: Exploring the Relationship between Eating and Intimacy* (New York: Dutton, 1991), Geneen Roth

13. *You Can Heal Your Life* (Santa Monica, CA: Hay

House, 1984) and *Life! Reflections on Your Journey* (Carlsbad, CA: Hay House, 1995), Louise L. Hay

14. *Reviving Ophelia: Saving the Selves of Adolescent Girls,* Mary Pipher, Ph.D. (New York: G. P. Putnam's Sons, 1994)

15. *Plus Style,* Suzan Nanfeldt (New York: Plume, 1996)

16. *Healing the Shame That Binds You,* John Bradshaw (Deerfield Beach, FL: Health Communications, Inc., 1988)

17. *The Power of Beauty,* Nancy Friday (New York: HarperCollins, 1996)

18. *Make the Connection: Ten Steps to a Better Body and a Better Life,* Bob Greene and Oprah Winfrey (New York: Hyperion, 1996)

Recommended Resources

The organizations below are the best I could find for questions on obesity, diet, compulsive eating disorders and related social issues. Let them help you.

American Anorexia/Bulimia Association
165 W. 46th Street
Suite 1108
New York, NY 10036
(212) 575-6200

Anorexia Nervosa and Related Eating Disorders, Inc.
P.O. Box 5102
Eugene, OR 97405
(541) 344-1144

Association for the Health Enrichment of Large
　People (AHELP)
P.O. Box Drawer C
Radford, VA 24142
(703) 731-1778

Center for Eating Disorders
North Shore University Hospital
444 Community Drive
Manhasset, NY 11030
(516) 869-6831

Eating Disorders Awareness and Prevention (EDAP)
603 Stewart Street
Suite 803
Seattle, WA 98101
(206) 382-3587

Largely Positive, Inc.
P.O. Box 17223
Glendale, WI 53217

National Association of Anorexia Nervosa and
　Associated Disorders (ANAD)
Box 7
Highland Park, IL 60035
(847) 831-3438

Recommended Resources

National Center for Overcoming Overeating
P.O. Box 1257
Old Chelsea Station
New York, NY 10011
(212) 875-0442

National Eating Disorders Organization (NEDO)
6655 South Yale Avenue
Tulsa, OK 74136
(918) 481-4044
This organization can refer you to clinics and doctors
in your area

P.L.E.A.S.E. (Promoting Legislation and Education
    About Self-Esteem)
91 South Main Street
West Hartford, CT 06107
(860) 521-2515
e-mail: PLEASE INC@aol.com

The Renfrew Foundation
475 Spring Lane
Philadelphia, PA 19128
(800) REN-FREW (736-3739)

Recommended Catalogue Shopping

Some of my most productive (and least painful) shopping sprees are conducted through the various catalogues that pile up in my mailbox each week. Below, you'll find some of my favorite large-size mail order companies. Call or write to them for a catalogue . . . and thank me later.

Alice's Undercover World
23820 Crenshaw Blvd.
Torrance, CA 90505
(310) 326-6775

Amplestuff
Dept. BG2, P.O. Box 116
Bearsville, NY 12409

Appleseeds
30 Tozer Road
Beverly, MA 01915
(800) 767-6666

Armand's
219X Elm Street
Reading, PA 19606

Avon by Mail
(800) 500-2866

Becoming Baby
Box 7238
Cumberland, RI 02864

Big, Bold & Beautiful
1263 Bay Street
Toronto, Ontario
Canada M5R 2C1
(800) 668-4673

Brownstone Woman
P.O. Box 2256
Salisbury, MD 21802
(800) 221-2468

Danskin Plus
(800) 288-6749

Essence by Mail
P.O. Box 62
Hanover, PA 17333
(800) 637-7362

Fit to Be Tried
4754 E. Grant
Tucson, AZ 85712
(520) 881-6449

Frederick's of Hollywood
P.O. Box 229
Hollywood, CA 90078
(800) 323-9525

Just My Size
P.O. Box 748
Rural Hall, NC 27098
Activewear: (800) 300-2600
Hosiery: (800) 522-0889

Peaches
P.O. Box 268
Cedarhurst, NY 11516
(800) PEACH03 (732-2403)

J. C. Penney
P.O. Box 2021
Milwaukee, WI 53201
(800) 222-6161

Roaman's
P.O. Box 46283
Indianapolis, IN 46209
(800) 274-7130

Sears
Woman's View Catalog
P.O. Box 8361
Indianapolis, IN 46283
(800) 944-1973

Silhouettes
5 Avery Road
Roanoke, VA 24012
(800) 704-3322

Recommended Catalogue Shopping

Spiegel For You
P.O. Box 182555
Columbus, OH 43218
(800) 345-4500

Ulla Popkin
825 Dulaney Valley Road
Towson Town Center
Towson, MD 21204
(800) 245-ULLA (8552)

Recommended Stores

I'd also like to give you the names of department and specialty stores that you can call for a location nearest you. Happy shopping! (They all have catalogues as well, so ask for one!)

August Max Woman
(800) 635-7500

Bloomingdale's Shop for Women
(212)705-3683

Bon Marché
(206) 344-2121

Burdines
(305) 835-5151

Charisma (NY and NJ only)
(800) 827-2427

Dayton Hudson
(612) 375-2200

Dillards
(501) 376-5200

Elisabeth of Liz Claiborne
(800) 555-9839 (press 1 for info)

Lane Bryant
Store location: (800) 888-9233
Mail order: (800) 477-7070

Lord & Taylor
American Women Dept.
(800) 223-7440

Macy's
(800) 343-0121

Nordstrom (Encore Dept.)
(800) 695-8000

Playtex Body Language
(888) GET-BODY (438-2639)

This is not a store, but an office
providing information on Playtex
undergarments.

Saks Fifth Avenue
Salon Z
(212) 753-4000

. . . .

Readers interested in contacting Emme
are encouraged to do so by writing to her
in care of her publisher:

The Putnam Berkley Group
200 Madison Avenue
New York, NY 10016

Or contact Emme through her Web site:
www.emmesupermodel.com